ALTERNATIVE MEDICINE

Alternative Medicine

Helpful or Harmful?

ROBINA COKER BSc MB BS MRCP (UK)

CHRISTIAN MEDICAL FELLOWSHIP

MONARCH
Crowborough

First British edition 1995

British Library Cataloguing in Publication Data
A catalogue record for this book is available
from the British Library.

ISBN: 1 85424 324 1

Designed and produced by
Bookprint Creative Services
P.O. Box 827, BN21 3YJ, England for
MONARCH PUBLICATIONS
Broadway House, The Broadway
Crowborough, E. Sussex TN6 1HQ.
Printed in Great Britain

CONTENTS

ACKNOWLEDGEMENTS

I should like to take this opportunity to thank the Christian Medical Fellowship for a grant from the Founders' Scholarship Fund which has helped me to write the book.

My heartfelt thanks go to Julia, Michael, Jennet, Barbara, Cathy, Gaz, Nick and Mike for their prayers and encouragement.

I am indebted to Mark Armstrong for supplying me with details of the work of the Medicines Control Agency.

Finally, I am very grateful to Andrew Fergusson for his patience and support throughout and for his helpful comments during the preparation of the manuscript.

Christian Medical Fellowship has well over 4,000 British doctors in all branches of the profession as members. It seeks to relate Christianity into the medical world, and medicine into the Christian world, and in partnership with others has a growing influence nationally and internationally.

For general enquiries contact:

Christian Medical Fellowship
157 Waterloo Road
London
SE1 8XN
Tel 0171-928 4694

CMF and the author regret that they cannot enter into correspondence concerning individual clinical queries.

FOREWORD

In 1984 I was an ordinary working GP, practising no alternative medicines—unless praying for patients, and occasionally with them, counts in this category! However, like many others, I was becoming increasingly aware of what some of my patients were getting interested in and I was forced to recognise the rise and rise of alternative medicine.

Because I had the privilege of sitting as an ordinary Christian Medical Fellowship member on its Medical Study Group, I took part between 1984 and 1985 in an extended investigation of the phenomenon, and that period opened my eyes in many ways. We listened first-hand to practitioners (most of whom were Christians) of different alternative therapies, we were sometimes amazed and sometimes amused, we heard for the first time about the 'New Age Movement' but above all we looked for explanations and reasons behind this popularity.

We realised that in recent years doctors have gained in the *science* of medicine at the expense of losing the *art*. I am sceptical that alternative medicines work in an objective sense, but I am not at all surprised that many of its practitioners bring relief. My patients didn't necessarily expect to get better, but they all wanted to feel better. Most GPs regularly ask a question like 'How are you in yourself?' and this is at least implicitly acknowledging that we should not just be technicians of cure, but concerned for the real needs of whole persons. Alternative medicine's popularity presents us with a much needed challenge to return to the art of healing. This at least has been helpful!

However, Dr Coker rightly reminds us in the words of the Bible: 'Test everything. Hold on to the good.' We dare not be uncritical. Alternative medicines can certainly be harmful physically and psychologically; I believe they can sometimes bring spiritual harm too.

We should always be concerned above all else with the *truth* of any issue—whether it be the truth or otherwise of the claims of Christianity, or of the claims of a particular alternative therapy. Unlike the New Ager, who believes 'everything is relative', and believes its corollary, 'there are no absolutes', the Christian and the scientist know that there is absolute truth. Some of that truth is knowable.

Enough is knowable for anyone to make a decision for or against Christianity. Unfortunately, not enough is necessarily knowable regarding the details of every individual alternative therapy, but this book provides the best approach yet available in the English language for assessing the truth or otherwise of the principles and practice of alternative medicine. Is it helpful or harmful? Read on and find out how to decide for yourself!

Andrew Fergusson BSc MB BS MRCGP
General Secretary, Christian Fellowship

Part I

INTRODUCTION

It is the glory of God to conceal a matter;
to search out a matter is the glory of kings.

Proverbs 25:2

For by him all things were created:

Colossians 1:16

Aims

In writing this book I have two broad aims, which divide
the book naturally into two sections. Firstly, I want to
explore some of the background to what is often called
alternative or complementary medicine.

In chapter one I have therefore included some definitions
so that we are clear what we are talking about. In chapter
two I have put both alternative and orthodox medicine in a
brief historical setting because I think this helps us to
understand the way medicine is practised in our society
today. In chapter three I have examined some of the
reasons underlying the current interest in alternative
therapies.

Secondly, I want to suggest some principles by which
we can examine all aspects of medicine more critically. I
hope that in this way we will be encouraged to develop

informed opinions about the various forms of medicine we encounter. Such information is crucial to an objective understanding of alternative medicine.

In chapter four I have outlined some of the problems which we encounter when dealing with alternative medicine. In chapter five I have examined how treatments can be evaluated objectively. In chapter six I have summarised ways in which we might use this information wisely to increase our knowledge and understanding of medicine.

Finally, in chapter seven I have partly yielded to the inevitable pressure to produce the definitive guide to all existing forms of alternative therapy. It is in reality neither definitive nor exhaustive, and the interested reader should look to other references for details.

The Christian Medical Fellowship

The Christian Medical Fellowship (CMF) is an association of doctors who believe in the truth of the Bible and in Jesus Christ as the Son of God. Although the opinions expressed in this book will probably not reflect those of all CMF members, we would agree that the Bible is an authoritative source of wisdom in the 20th century and that conventional western medicine is a reasonable yardstick with which to compare alternative practices. This philosophy therefore underlies this book.

Christianity and Science

Such an approach is open to several criticisms. Many people today assume that science has replaced the Bible. Some may therefore argue that the Christian faith is just as empirical (that is, knowledge is derived from experience rather than from scientific proof) as the practices of alternative medicine under consideration, and should therefore not be used as a reference point. Others may claim that conventional medicine has often failed in its attempts to promote the health of society, and should not be regarded as an ideal standard with which to compare other forms of therapy.

Finally, the Christian faith and scientific reasoning may be held to be incompatible. The Church has in the past sometimes branded scientists as heretics. The most notable example is probably that of Galileo who was forced by the Inquisition to recant his support of the Copernican system. This stated that the earth and the planets rotated round the sun, for us today an accepted fact in the life of our universe.

Others would consider that the whole process of faith (that is, believing without seeing) is irreconcilable with the basis of science, which involves testing hypotheses and accepting only those facts for which there exists objective proof.

However, I think these criticisms can be answered. Firstly, there exists a wealth of apologetics for the Christian faith derived from objective historical evidence, available for anyone who wishes to study it. The reader could begin with Nicky Gumbel's *Questions of Life*[1] for a general introduction, or Josh McDowell's *Evidence That Demands A Verdict* for a more detailed study.[2] Christianity is thus not exclusively based on subjective or personal experience.

Secondly, biblical principles for living are in fact not as outdated as some may think. Take as an example the sixth of the Ten Commandments: 'You shall not murder'.[3] I wonder how many people would really contest this as a general principle for society. I am deliberately not going to begin to discuss war, capital punishment, abortion or euthanasia.

One bleak day in February 1993 in Bootle, Liverpool, two ten-year-old boys tortured and murdered a toddler. His name was James Bulger, and his murder will probably be remembered as one of the most notable crimes in British history. At the trial the judge said that the murder had been an evil act. I don't think anyone would actually dispute that statement, although the causes of and the responsibility for such evil are undoubtedly less easy to define and will remain open to debate for all time.

Thirdly, although it is impossible either to prove or disprove the existence of God using scientific methods, so that their application to this end is unrewarding, God has given mankind the gifts of wisdom and understanding, and these include scientific discoveries. This should come as no surprise to us if we view science as one means of discovering more about the physical properties of the world that God created.

Western medicine is now firmly rooted in scientific principles and research. This does not justify its failings, which reflect instead our imperfect understanding. It is however reasonable to use the scientific principles and research which are the foundations of Western medicine to evaluate new therapeutic approaches.

Amongst other things the Bible upholds truth, honesty, compassion and justice. These are acknowledged to be important principles in medicine. Doctors are required to be honest with their patients and most are also compassionate. Medical scientists are required to be truthful in their research. Justice in medicine surely means ensuring equal access to equal healthcare for all, regardless of colour, sex, age or financial status. Christians can therefore be confident that the Bible's message is relevant for society in the 20th and 21st centuries.

Who Is This Book For?

I have written this book with the general reader in mind and have therefore devoted some space to explaining medical terms and principles where they are important to the discussion. Church members not infrequently ask me what I think about acupuncture or homoeopathy, although they do not always get a sensible answer! I hope this book will help them to understand the standpoint of much of the medical profession and to clarify their own views.

However, I hope that some of the ideas expressed here will interest a wider audience. Many in the healthcare professions are concerned by the increased popularity of alternative medicine and wish to preserve the practice of medicine based on established scientific principles and accurate research. A more specific readership, that of Christian doctors and medical students, is also envisaged.

What This Book Is Not

This book is not an authoritative or exhaustive guide to all the forms of alternative medicine being practised today, either in this country or abroad. The field of alternative medicine is expanding so rapidly that such a guide would be outdated before publication.

The converse is also true, with practices until very recently considered unorthodox now being included in more conventional medical practice. A notable example is that of osteopathy. The Osteopaths Act, which became law on 1 July 1993, made osteopathy the first branch of alternative medicine to be formally recognised and regulated in the United Kingdom. Another example is acupuncture, now frequently offered by anaesthetists alongside traditional treatment in pain clinics and intensive care units.

Instead I have tried to examine the principles behind both alternative and conventional medicine from biblical and scientific perspectives. I hope this will challenge us to look honestly and carefully at any new practice we encounter. Ultimately I hope that more of the truth about alternative medicine can be discovered, and a scientific and equitable approach to healthcare in this country maintained.

Why Write This Book?

To some Christians this book may seem superfluous. Many see our country as being in the grip of a crisis of lawlessness, violence and marital breakdown. I referred to the murder of two-year-old James Bulger in 1993 by two ten-year-old boys, themselves apparently emotionally deprived. This appalling event, felt by many as a dreadful indictment of British society today, left almost nobody untouched. The roles of Church and government in the moral welfare of society are being challenged.

Christians may therefore feel there are more pressing issues to consider than whether it is wrong to indulge in a little aromatherapy when slightly unwell. 'After all, it may not work, but it's pretty harmless isn't it?' However, I hope to show that the issue of alternative medicine is of importance. Some of the questions raised in this book can be applied to other aspects of contemporary life. Finding answers to these may help us to understand more clearly how we as individuals can influence both the present and future of the society in which we live.

There are several specific reasons why the CMF has felt that the issue of alternative medicine should be discussed.

Rising Demand and Practice

Demand

The popularity and public awareness of alternative forms of therapy have grown greatly in the last twenty years in Britain. A 1986 survey suggested that approximately 15% of people in Britain consulted alternative practitioners.[4]

Recently published data assembled from surveys performed between 1985 and 1992 show that 26% of the population in this country use at least one form of alternative therapy.[5]

Further breakdown of these figures reveals that 36% have received manipulation (including osteopathic or chiropractic), 24% have had recourse to phytotherapy (plant-based treatment) or herbalism and 16% have received acupuncture or homoeopathy. Furthermore, an impressive 74% of the British public apparently favour alternative therapy being available on the National Health Service (NHS).

The rising interest in alternative medicine is not confined to this country. In 1992 about 60% of the German population used alternative therapy.[6] In 1981 only 6% of the Dutch population used alternative remedies but by 1990 this figure had risen to 16%. Use of homoeopathy in France has more than doubled in ten years, increasing from 16% in 1982 to 36% in 1992.[7] In the United States, 34% of the population have recourse to alternative forms of therapy.

Alternative medicine in Britain has also received support in parliamentary circles. In 1989 the Parliamentary Group for Alternative and Complementary Medicine was established, serving as a political focus for the alternative medicine lobby.

Practice

It has always been difficult to ascertain with accuracy the number of non-conventional therapists in the UK. This is because there are no comprehensive registers. However, the following figures serve as a rough pointer to the growing practice of alternative medicine. To take just one example, the number of professional acupuncturists reportedly doubled between 1978 and 1981.[8]

A 1987 survey estimated that there were at least 1900

practitioners of acupuncture, chiropractic, homoeopathy, naturopathy and osteopathy in Britain.[9] However, in 1991 a survey conducted by the British Medical Association (BMA) reported that there were at least 3000 osteopaths and acupuncturists alone.[10] Since the early 1980s there has been an estimated three-fold increase in the number of practising osteopaths who now treat approximately 100,000 patients each week.[11] In Germany in 1992 over 30% of general practitioners and hospital specialists pre-scribed alternative remedies.[12] Reflecting an even more striking change in medical opinion, in 1990 over 20% of general practitioners in the Netherlands considered that acupuncture is an effective treatment for asthma.[13]

Even by the early 1980s the medical profession could no longer ignore this wave of enthusiasm. In 1983 the BMA established a working party on alternative therapy to examine the claims made for these therapies. Their aims were twofold: to discover whether potentially useful meth-ods of treatment were being ignored, and whether false claims of benefit were being made. These questions remain of crucial importance. A full national survey of non-conventional therapies was conducted by the BMA in 1991 and the results published in 1993.[14]

As recent articles in the British Medical Journal (BMJ) demonstrate,[15] individual doctors are also increasingly being challenged to voice their opinions about the surge in unorthodox treatments. Many of their own patients may be seeking alternative remedies and using these in addition to, or instead of, drugs prescribed by their doctor. Given the possible deleterious consequences on patients' obser-vance of their doctor's instructions, and the risks of drug toxicity, this has implications for all doctors involved in patient care regardless of whether they choose to partici-pate in the public debate.

The wave of enthusiasm has even reached petcare! Several central London veterinary clinics now routinely

offer homoeopathy. One manufacturer of pet foods adver-
tises its products as being 'in accord with nature' and
promotes a wide range of herbal and other alternative
medicines, including cod liver oil capsules, elderberry,
garlic, raspberry, rhubarb and seaweed tablets and wheat-
germ oil capsules. A 'natural diet' is recommended 'to
ensure your pet enjoys the healthy lifestyle it deserves'.
Does this sound familiar?

Medical Education

The rise in alternative medicine has implications for medical education. Our opinions and decisions will ultimately
mould those of succeeding generations of doctors. Already
some forms of alternative medicine, for example aromatherapy, are being introduced into hospital settings
and medical students will increasingly be confronted with
them. There are plans to introduce alternative medicine
into the medical school curriculum in at least one university.[16] If the undergraduate medical curriculum changes, so
may the boundaries of orthodox medical practice.

We have a responsibility to teach medical students to
apply constructive criticism to the subjects they are taught,
and to be ready to challenge new developments if appropriate. The critical study of unorthodox remedies provides
an excellent model for teaching medical students the
principles of evaluation of any new therapy, conventional
or otherwise. It is obviously essential to good medical
practice and cost-effectiveness to try to ensure that all
remedies offered to the public are safe and effective.

European Laws

In a broader context, European Union (EU) legislation
over the next few years may well limit some of these
practices. The general public seems largely unaware that

Britain is unusual in allowing lay practitioners consider-able freedom, so that the practice of alternative medicine in this country is virtually unregulated. In most other European countries only registered health professionals are allowed to offer alternative therapies. In future, EU harmonisation of the training and regulation of alternative practitioners may be required. The unregulated practice of alternative therapists could then be outlawed. We need to have a clear idea of what we consider to be good medicine if we are to ensure that appropriate laws, protecting the interests of patients, are passed.

The Christian Debate

Christians believe in one sovereign God, and they believe that He is embodied in the person of Jesus Christ. For them the implications of alternative remedies, some founded on other spiritual beliefs and practices, may cause concern. However, in order to respond wisely it is imperative that Christians know the facts first, or they could generate needless fear and prohibitions.

Within the church, the recently revitalised interest in healing, particularly within more charismatic sectors, has brought a renewed quest for health. Unorthodox remedies may consequently be sampled in addition to more conven-tional ones. Ironically perhaps, prayer for healing may be regarded by some outside the church as just another form of alternative therapy. The church may need to consider this seriously if it is to avoid bans on public prayer of this kind.

Christians may be critical of mass healing meetings such as the Morris Cerullo healing rallies held in London in June 1992, August 1993 and August 1994. However, we must realise that all so-called healing ministries could potentially be viewed with equal scepticism by those outside the church. Whilst this book does not set out to discuss the issue of 'healing' in the church today, this issue obviously affects the way many Christians view modern medicine. Christian leaders need to be open enough to discuss these issues and ready to apply their biblical knowledge to such situations in a way which will honour God and benefit their congregations.

Few Guidelines

Finally, there are relatively few books written on the subject in this country. The BMA's recent publication[17] and 'Alternative Medicine in Britain'[18] help fill gaps in the medical and social scientific literature but still leave room for the views of Christian doctors to be heard.

WHAT IS ALTERNATIVE MEDICINE?

A faithful friend is the medicine of life

Ecclesiasticus 6:16

He is before all things,
and in him all things hold together

Colossians 1:17

What is Health?

In order to understand what lies behind alternative medicine, we need to define what we mean by health. This is more complex than it may seem initially, as the following discussion makes clear.

The Collins Concise English Dictionary defines health as 'the state of being bodily and mentally vigorous and free of disease'. This definition excludes concepts of health in terms of relationships between individuals or of spiritual health.

The World Health Organisation goes one step further by defining health as 'a state of complete physical, mental and social well-being and not merely as the absence of illness or disease'. This definition still excludes the concept of spiritual health, because it gives no credence to the idea that there is a God who intervenes in the affairs of mankind. It may also be interpreted somewhat unrealistically as suggesting that it is possible to live in this world completely without pain, suffering or conflict in communities.

A fuller discussion of possible definitions of health from a Christian viewpoint has been presented by David Atkinson.[1] The author starts with Jesus Christ as his reference point in deciding what constitutes a healthy human being. From the creation story recorded in the opening chapters of Genesis, the first book of the Bible, he shows that God intended human life to be lived in a satisfying physical environment in companionship with other human beings as well as in a fulfilling relationship with Himself.

The most casual observer of human life on this planet cannot fail to note that this ideal has not been achieved. Christians explain this situation as resulting from the effects of sin. Sin can be defined simply as any offence against a principle or standard. Christians define sin more specifically as any transgression of standards established by God. This includes all rebellion against God. The Bible teaches that the effect of sin is to shatter human beings' relationships with God and to distort people's relationships with each other. Wider evidence of the consequences of sin can be seen in the crime and injustice that corrupt human society and in the devastation of our environment.

One theme running through the Old Testament is the way in which people fail to measure up to God's standards. However, the Bible does not stop here. In the New Testament it teaches that God has dealt with sin by offering forgiveness in Jesus Christ. When God forgives sins, He does not ignore them or lightly dismiss human guilt. Instead, God considers the death of Jesus Christ through crucifixion as a sacrifice which pays for the sins of humankind. Those individuals who accept God's offer of forgiveness also receive a new life which gives them the freedom to choose to reject sinful behaviour and obey God's principles instead.

It follows that the work of God in Christians who have received His forgiveness will include dealing with the effects of sin in their lives. The word 'salvation' is used biblically to symbolise this deliverance of God's people from sinful actions and their consequences. Salvation includes physical, psychological and spiritual healing. Such healing is illustrated by Jesus Christ's works while on this earth and described in the historical accounts of His life known as the Gospels. The restoration of relation-ships between men and women, and between mankind and the environment is alluded to later in the New Testament, in a collection of letters written to young churches and known as the Epistles.

However, the New Testament also makes it clear that healing in all its fullness is not promised until the estab-lishment of a new heaven and a new earth. David Atkinson concludes that the Bible views health as a holistic concept which includes 'individual and social, physical and men-tal, temporal and spiritual life', and he is clear that whole-ness of this kind can only ever be partial in this life.

There will be those who would prefer to ignore a spiritual dimension to health on the basis that it is unscien-tific to do so. Such readers might consider that there are psychiatrists who will testify to recognising the existence of forces of evil which they had not previously believed in. Some have subsequently reconsidered the possibility of the existence of God. Others have gone further and claimed that a spiritual dimension is essential if modern psychiatry is to understand fully human nature and behaviour.

One such is Dr Scott Peck. He writes: 'In common with 99 per cent of psychiatrists . . . I did not think the devil existed. Still, priding myself on being an open-minded scientist, I felt I had to examine the evidence . . . So I decided to go out and look for a case [of demon possession]. Referrals trickled in. The first two cases turned out to be suffering from standard psychiatric disorders, as I had suspected, and I began making marks on my scientific pistol. The third case turned out to be the real thing . . . I now know Satan is real. I have met it.'[2]

That health should have a spiritual dimension should not really come as a surprise to us, even in the 20th century. After all, science sheds no real light on questions of purpose or morality. No doubt all of us will at some stage in our lives wonder why we are here and what our purpose is, or why there is so much pain and suffering in the world. Answers to 'spiritual' questions such as these are not readily found in the study of science, but rather in the spiritual realm.

What is Medicine?

Having attempted to define health, we need to consider definitions of medicine. The Collins Concise English Dictionary defines medicine as 'any drug or remedy for use in treating, preventing or alleviating the symptoms of disease'. This obviously covers both medicine and surgery. If we accept the holistic definition of health given above, this definition will be seen to be too narrow, since it excludes the concepts of social health and spiritual well-being. However, for the present discussion I will use the dictionary definition of medicine as a working basis. I have chosen to do this because it is the concept with which doctors, nurses, physiotherapists and other health-care professionals are most concerned.

What is Alternative Medicine?

Even using a fairly narrow definition of medicine, alternative medicine is surprisingly difficult to define. Consequently the definition is sometimes rather arbitrarily made on the basis of personal beliefs. Some have included disciplines regarded by the majority of the medical profession as part of recognised medical practice.

For instance, one Christian writer has included psychotherapy among his list of alternative therapies.[3] Closer reading reveals that he is writing from the perspective of someone previously involved in spiritualism who is rightly concerned lest others fall into a similar trap through any of the plethora of so-called 'psychological therapies' available outside the NHS. However, psychotherapy has been available on the NHS for many years and is part of the range of treatments available to the psychiatrist.

That psychotherapy is accepted as part of conventional medicine does not necessarily mean that it has been proved to be effective. There is evidence that some conditions such as depression and anxiety respond better to drugs combined with psychotherapy than to drugs alone and some studies have shown psychological treatments to be more effective than no treatment at all.[4] However, not all studies have been well-designed to answer the question they are asking, and some have shown little or no differences in outcome with psychotherapy.

However, the inclusion of psychotherapy in standard medical practice does mean that for the purposes of this book I will not include it in the category of 'alternative' medicine.

It is obvious that if we use personal preferences to decide whether a treatment is acceptable two different people may reach quite different conclusions, even when they share the Christian faith. For example, someone else, concerned about possible side-effects associated with powerful drugs, might regard psychotherapy for the treatment of chronic depression as being preferable to that of antidepressants. Some other means of evaluation, preferably objective, must therefore be chosen. Objective evaluation of treatments, including the use of clinical trials, is discussed in chapter five.

Some medical and surgical practice has been fully validated by scientific evidence and clinical trials. However, the British government has in recent years emphasised the importance of 'audit' in the NHS. Audit is a term originally used to describe inspection and verification of business accounts by an accountant. In the context of the NHS it describes the examination and comparison of current medical and surgical procedures with a previously established standard. This is usually done at the level of individual departments within hospitals and can include such diverse topics as the quality of medical records, implementation of procedures carried out during an emergency (for example a cardiac arrest) or the time spent by junior doctors performing administrative or nursing tasks. It may result in hospital guidelines being drawn up and local practices being altered.

As a consequence, healthcare professionals, hospital managers and the general public are becoming increasingly aware that a number of apparently well-established and effective treatments have never been subjected to objective scrutiny. It is therefore impracticable to define alternative medicine as those therapies not proven to be effective by clinical trials.

The Medical School Curriculum

For simplicity I shall therefore define alternative medicine as all 'medical' practice not currently included within the medical curriculum, orthodox medicine comprising those subjects with which medical students may reasonably be expected to be familiar before becoming fully qualified doctors.

The medical curriculum at present requires students to acquire a working knowledge of the basic medical sciences (anatomy, biochemistry, physiology, pharmacology, psychology and sociology) as well as an understanding of the principles and practice of the different branches of medicine and surgery. These comprise medicine (including all the branches of hospital medicine, examples being cardiology and dermatology, and the field of general practice), surgery (including general surgery and specialties such as ear, nose and throat surgery and plastic surgery), obstetrics and gynaecology, paediatrics (medicine in children and the newborn) and basic psychiatry.

This is not a perfect definition, but has the merits of being familiar to medical readers and reasonably objective.

Holistic or Complementary?

'Holistic' and 'complementary' are other terms frequently used synonymously with 'alternative' medicine. I have deliberately chosen to use the term alternative medicine.

The expression 'holistic' merely means that in treating disease, consideration is given to the complete person. In routine medical practice this should include a brief and informal assessment of the patient's intelligence and personality, their understanding of, and attitude towards, their illness, and some insight into their financial and social resources. It should also include a thorough assessment of any other medical conditions and medications they may already be receiving.

Medical students are introduced to these principles throughout their clinical course and the skills needed to perform such an assessment are gradually acquired during subsequent years. Within the limitations of the busy NHS, such an assessment should therefore be part of good medical practice and not the prerogative of alternative practitioners. Such considerations are in any case essential for the doctor to decide on the most appropriate treatment and help ensure that the patient is able to receive it.

Furthermore, certain alternative therapies, such as osteopathy, apply a mechanistic rather than holistic approach to disease. This means that, in treating back pain, the primary concern of the osteopath is to restore correct function to the musculoskeletal system while emphasising the role of physical treatment. Although a good osteopath will enquire about emotional and psychological stresses in the patient's life, which may for example alter the patient's attitude to pain or disability, there is no reason to suppose that the outlook of the osteopath is any more holistic than that of a caring and competent general practitioner. That the word holistic has come to be synonymous with alternative medicine is to some extent an indictment of orthodox medicine, as we shall see later.

The 'complementary' label implies that orthodox medicine is in itself incomplete. This is undoubtedly true, partly because there remain many scientific and therapeutic advances to be made and partly because all doctors are human, and therefore, regrettably fallible. However, there are several reasons why I am disinclined to use this term.

Firstly, it has been shown that some substances present in herbal remedies are not harmless but in fact quite toxic. Evidence for this is discussed in chapter four. Since these substances have not been subjected to safety tests, such side-effects are unpredictable and may therefore in some circumstances be extremely dangerous. I therefore think it is only prudent to restrict the use of the word 'complementary' to those therapies which have been formally evaluated, both for efficacy and safety, along the lines described above.

Secondly, some therapies such as homoeopathy are based on principles which conflict fundamentally with those underlying orthodox medicine. This can be illustrated briefly as follows.

The basic mechanisms by which orthodox pharmaceutical agents exert their effects are generally known, at least in outline. A drug has to interact with a molecule (usually a protein) in the body before it can produce a therapeutic effect. It may bind to a specific receptor (a molecule, typically on a cell membrane, which 'recognises' the drug) or it may interact with a biological catalyst (an enzyme) responsible for controlling a biochemical reaction in a cell. This interaction leads to an alteration in cellular function. If the cell belongs to the organism and if sufficient drug molecules are present this will then lead to alteration in tissue and subsequently organ function.

Alternatively, if the cell targeted by the drug is a foreign one, such as a bacterial cell, bacterial function will be altered and the bacterium will ultimately die. Owing to the way drugs work, their pharmacological effects are related to their concentration at the site of action. Within certain limits, the higher the concentration, the greater is the resulting pharmacological effect. This 'dose-response relationship' is well established for drugs currently on the market, and is the basis of normal prescribing practice.

The practice of homoeopathy is based on entirely different principles. The active ingredient in homoeopathic remedies is diluted in an inactive vehicle such as water or alcohol until no molecule of the original active compound remains. According to the rational approach described above there is no reason to suppose that the active ingredient can be effective, since it is no longer physically present. However, homoeopathic practitioners believe that by subjecting this solution, now consisting only of the vehicle, to a series of shakes, called succussions, it becomes more potent.

These claims run completely contrary to the principles underlying modern drug therapy. It is therefore not possi-

ble to reconcile them in the light of our present understanding or to consider homoeopathy as being complementary to orthodox medicine.

It has been argued that since 'complementary practitioners' are not capable of making a careful diagnosis,
they should always work alongside orthodox medical
practitioners who will make the diagnosis and then refer
for treatment.[5] The term 'alternative' is thought to be ill-
conceived and 'complementary' more appropriate. However, I believe that this underestimates the quite competent
diagnosis that, for example, a chiropractor is able to reach
following a careful history and clinical examination.

The expression 'alternative' in my view accurately
summarises the standing of such therapies at present. In
some cases they may become complementary to orthodox
medicine, but only after rigorous evaluation.

What is 'The New Age'?

This is not a book about the New Age. However, the
Collins Concise English Dictionary defines New Age as
'a late 1980s philosophy characterised by a belief in
alternative medicine, astrology, spiritualism, etc.' No
discussion of alternative medicine can therefore be complete without a reference to the New Age.

The phrase 'New Age' was coined at the beginning of
this century by Annie Besant. She later became the leader
of the Theosophical Society which was founded in 1875
and embraced beliefs derived from the sacred writings of
Brahmanism and Buddhism. The expression 'New Age' is
derived from the astrological theory that each 'star-age'
lasts for 2000 years. Adherents of the New Age philosophy claim that we are now leaving the age of Pisces, the
fish, a sign identified with Christianity, and are entering
the age of Aquarius, identified with humanism.

Key tenets of this philosophy include pantheism – all

that exists is god, and so, by implication, we are all gods –
and relative rather than absolute morality – good and evil
are only illusions, therefore each individual must decide
his or her own morality. Shirley Maclaine is today one of
the best known protagonists of the New Age philosophy.

The contrast with Christianity is obvious. As outlined
earlier, Christians believe that there is one God who is
distinct from the world He created and that man is sepa-
rated from God by sin. Sin is an unpopular word today, but
everyone recognises selfish anger, lust, envy, hatred and
arrogant pride. These are some of the sins condemned in
the Bible. Reconciliation with God can only come through
faith in Jesus Christ, who said of Himself, 'I am the way
and the truth and the life. No-one comes to the Father
except through me'.[6]

God has given His people fundamental principles for
living. These are outlined in the Old Testament, in the text
we now know as the Ten Commandments.[7] Over 1400
years later they were summarised by Jesus as 'Love the
Lord your God with all your heart, and with all your soul
and with all your mind', and 'Love your neighbour as
yourself'.[8]

Not all alternative therapies are linked to the New Age
movement, but the quest for self-perfection and ever-
increasing health follows naturally from this philosophy.
New Age thinking incorporates astrology, magic and
crystal gazing. The belief that healing forces can be
harnessed through crystals and pyramids is also promoted. A number of alternative therapies do have their
roots in New Age thinking. It is because of considerations
such as these that Christians oppose the New Age movement and many are critical of alternative medicine.

However, I believe it is unwise to dismiss all such
treatments too hastily. The truth must in each case be
sought. It is also important to realise that the so-called
New Age philosophy is in fact anything but new: panthe-

ism, astrology and rejection of the concept of absolute morality can be traced back to antiquity. The Christian faith has survived 2000 years of heresies and persecutions. Christians need to remember this when considering alternative therapies. We can be confident in our God and we are invited to ask Him for wisdom when ours seems lacking.[9]

2

A HISTORICAL PERSPECTIVE

Whatever is has already been,
and what will be has been before.

Ecclesiastes 3:15

All professions are conspiracies against the laity.

George Bernard Shaw

Why History?

In chapter one we defined alternative medicine as comprising treatments currently not included in the medical school curriculum, and therefore existing outside the context of orthodox medicine. It follows from this definition that alternative medicine cannot be considered in isolation from orthodox medicine.

In our search for the background to alternative medicine we therefore need to explore the historical background to orthodox medicine. I believe this is important if we are to gain a clearer idea of the origins of both orthodox and alternative therapies and so put them in perspective.

The following historical sketch is of necessity a condensed outline. I have started by considering the origins of medicine throughout the world. I have then focused on medicine in Europe and in particular Britain. For more detailed accounts the interested reader may like to consult other references[1-4] from which this information is derived.

Primitive Societies

A feature common to all primitive cultures is to regard religion, magic and medical therapy as inseparable. The history of medicine has always been closely connected with that of religion because both have a similar aim: the defence of the individual against evil forces. Thus medicine has its origins largely in magical and religious practices. Primitive dances are quoted as an example of this. They were frequently part of complex rites in which the aid of supernatural forces was invoked. A witch-doctor prayed to the good gods and the dancers joined hands to form a chain as a token of protection from evil and sickness.

Primitive healers sought supernatural origins for most events including sickness. Sorcerers typically formed an exclusive caste in order to safeguard their secrets and heighten their authority. Consequently they usually occupied a high place socially and politically.

Magical medicine thus developed from largely empirical practices. Some magical practices worked because they depended on suggestion. Examples include spells and amulets, the latter worn to keep illness and evil spirits at bay. However, some practices are of relevance to modern medicine because they were based on the study of the healing properties of plants and the toxicity of animal poisons. Antidotes to snake venom were initially derived from such studies.

The Sumerian Civilisation

The Sumerian civilisation is the oldest civilisation of whose medicine we have knowledge. It was established in the southern region of Babylonia before the biblical

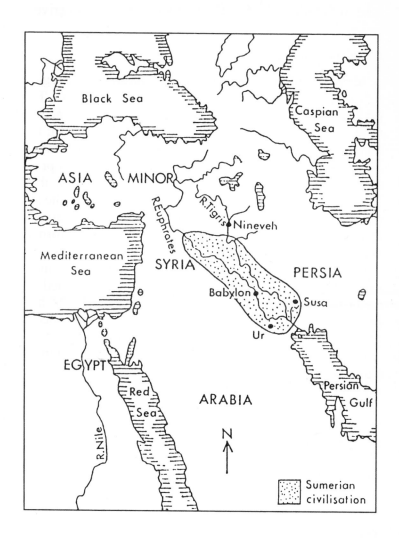

The Sumerian Civilisation
(Adapted from The Times Concise Atlas of World History. Times
Books Ltd: UK, 1982.)

time of Abraham (see map p. 39). The Sumerians based their medical practice on the study of astronomy (the study of stars and seasons) and later on astrology (the belief that man's destiny is subject to the stars). This civilisation waned about 2000 BC when it was absorbed by the Assyrians and Babylonians who conquered Mesopotamia.

The Assyrians and Babylonians

The Assyrio-Babylonians believed that disease was caused by demons, and astronomy remained central to their medical practice. It was held that only doctor-priests could interpret demonic actions and invoke the help of the gods. Answerable to the gods, these early medical practitioners nevertheless used many drugs derived from plants and animals and recognised various fevers, plagues, rheumatism, venereal diseases and tuberculosis. Much of their practice seems to have been a mixture of ritual and commonsense. For example, a drink of beer and sliced onion was prescribed for eye trouble. The use of onion is logical since it induces the flow of tears which contain lysozyme, an antibacterial agent. The Assyrio-Babylonian doctor-priests were highly regarded and often summoned to provide medical services as far away as Egypt.

In contrast to their medical colleagues, Assyrio-Babylonian surgeons were by 1900 BC developing professional status and were answerable to the civil authorities. King Hammurabi, king of Babylonia from about 1948 to 1905 BC, was the promulgator of one of the earliest known statutes of law, the code of King Hammurabi. Established in this were scales of fees and penalties for incompetence and negligence by surgeons.

The Egyptians

The Egyptians appear to have had quite a sophisticated national health service. The sick were treated free of charge in wartime and while on journeys, and doctors were paid by the State. There was also a high degree of specialisation amongst doctors. At a national level there was an emphasis on hygiene in dwellings, diet, sexual relations and burial. Respiration was considered vital and it was thought that circulation depended on breathing. Complaints of the heart, including angina, and abdominal and eye disorders were recognised, as were various swellings.

In about 420 BC Herodotus gives the following account of medicine practised in the Nile valley. '. . . each physician applies himself to one disease and not more. All places abound in physicians; some are for the eyes, others for the head, others for the teeth, others for the intestines and others for internal disorders'.[5]

Ancient India

In the highly structured society of India, doctors likewise occupied a clear niche. Medical works were grouped together in large collections resembling encyclopedias. It is consequently impossible to date them or identify the sources of ideas found in them. However, it is notable that surgery was especially advanced, particularly plastic surgery. Rhinoplasty, the reshaping of the nose, was frequently performed, since the nose was cut off as punishment for adultery. Diagnostic techniques were also quite advanced. For example, it was known that malaria is caused by mosquitoes. Brahmin regulations laid emphasis on personal hygiene and sanitation.

China

As in other cultures, Chinese medicine can be partly understood in the context of religious beliefs. In the Taoist legend of the creation of the world, creation occurred when chaos was overcome under the inspiration of the god Pan Ku and order established on the basis of two opposite poles, yang and yin. Yang represents the positive, active, masculine: left-handed, light, sky, dryness and warmth. Yin represents the negative, passive, feminine: right-handed, earth, moisture and cold. It was believed that illness resulted from an imbalance between these two poles.

The emperors influenced the development of medicine and initiated the most typically Chinese practice, that of acupuncture. Herbal remedies were well known. They included the use of opium as a narcotic, rhubarb as a laxative, and ephedrine (derived from the stem of the Chinese herb ephedra) for asthma. Iron was given to treat anaemia, kaolin for diarrhoea, and the first steps were taken to immunise against smallpox.

Japan

Little is known of early Japanese medicine. In the fourth century AD Chinese civilisation penetrated Japan and for many centuries its medicine supplanted native remedies. The Portuguese landing in 1542 introduced European medical practices which were adopted as avidly as the Chinese ones before them.

The Hebrews

The biblical Hebrews seem to have inherited a number of their beliefs from ancient Mesopotamian culture, among them the conviction that disease was divine punishment and a mark of sin. However, in contrast to Egypt and Mesopotamia, the monotheistic Hebrews viewed God as their true healer. Belief in one god excluded the use of magical practices. Resorting to divination, omens, exorcists or sorcerers was forbidden by law[6] and was abhorrent to God. Physical and moral purity were equated, and the Jews were notable in that regulations regarding hygiene were applied to the entire people and not merely to the priests or certain castes as in other primitive societies.

The belief that disease was the outcome of sin was later passed on to Christian medieval Europe. Although the Bible teaches that some diseases do indeed result from sin, there are also many instances where the Bible makes it clear that disease and suffering generally occur for other reasons, some not fully explained. The book of Job in the Old Testament and Jesus' own teaching are examples of this.[7,8]

The Greeks

Hellenic medicine is unique in the ancient world because it developed alongside a philosophy disciplined by strict criticism. For the first time, healing became a science as well as an art. Magic was gradually replaced by enquiry and came to be regarded as a noble science.

From the sixth century BC onwards, attempts were emerging to give all phenomena natural rather than supernatural explanations. Medicine in Greece gradually acquired professional status. Schools of medicine were established and pupils had to apply for a licence to practise, which was only given when the standing of the school they attended had been taken into account. Practitioners were allowed to open surgeries and treat patients for fees. Army and gymnasium doctors (the latter comparable to the sports physicians of today) were also licensed.

The medical school which was to become the most

famous was that on the island of Kos. Its teaching emphasised the importance of physical examination and diagnosis. Prognosis (the opinion of the probable course and outcome of an illness) and aetiology (the science of the investigation of the cause or origin of disease) were also studied and taught.

Hippocrates was born on the island of Kos about 460 BC and learnt from his father. By this time medical practitioners no longer regarded illness as punishment by the gods but instead sought rational methods of treatment. Hippocrates travelled widely and taught that suffering could be relieved by hygiene and proven cures, not by help from magic.

Hippocrates was at the forefront of medical science in his time and attempted to classify knowledge under the headings of anatomy, physiology, general pathology, diagnosis, therapy, prognosis, surgery, obstetrics and gynaecology, mental illness and ethics. His rational approach represented a huge advance in medical thinking.

The concept of the four basic humours of the body (blood, phlegm, yellow bile and black bile) was also developed around this time, and illness attributed to an imbalance of one of these. If this idea strikes us as ludicrous, we should perhaps remember that it was still regarded as valid until the first half of the 19th century.

Hellenic culture extended through the Aegean and Ionian islands to the coasts of Asia Minor, reaching Italy and Sicily. Greek practitioners after Hippocrates gradually infiltrated Rome. The Roman view was that medicine was supernatural and magical and they were too proud to practise medicine, believing that such practice was only appropriate for slaves. However, the extension of Greek culture gradually changed this attitude.

In later Greek culture, Oriental influences grew more important and medicine became increasingly associated with religion. Literature after Homer illustrates this in that it contains numerous references to incantations, demons, omens and soothsayers.

Europe and The Arabs

The fall of Rome in AD 476 probably resulted from a combination of private and public corruption, oppression of minorities and incursions by barbarians. In the ensuing disorder, rational thought became impossible. The dissolution of the Roman institutions of law and medicine followed, and nonclerical physicians ceased to exist. Epidemics of bubonic plague raged through the empire and individuals, rendered powerless in the face of these new enemies, turned again to magic for deliverance and relief.

In the chaos of wars and plagues which covered Europe in the Middle Ages, the welfare of the sick was taken over by religious orders. Nuns and monks were never involved in fighting and so were the only people who enjoyed the detachment and peace necessary to care for the wounded and the sick. Monasteries thus provided much of the available medical care, which was therefore controlled by the church. Infirmaries were built in the monasteries and medicines made from plants growing in the grounds.

A different situation existed in the world of Islam, where Greco-Roman knowledge was translated and preserved. The Arabic peoples (including dispersed Christians, Persians and Jews) established pharmacy and chemistry as sciences, built hospitals and developed knowledge of such diseases as tuberculosis. Training institutions for physicians flourished and in the tenth century the caliph of Baghdad required that all practitioners take an examination before being licensed.

Orthodox European medical education was later developed in the newly established universities. The most renowned school of medicine came into being in Salerno in Italy in the tenth century and reached its height of fame in the late 11th century. Founded on Greek, Latin and Islamic civilisations in the ninth century, it was free of clerical control and, remarkably, open to female practitioners. In 1240 Frederick II granted it the right to license doctors to practise. No one could work as a physician unless authorised. Permission was given after a five year course of study and one year of practice under expert supervision. From Salerno originated a collection of celebrated prescriptions, the parent of subsequent pharmacopoeias. Salerno also retained many Hippocratic aphorisms and teachings were put into verse so that they could be easily remembered. The influence of the Salerno school later spread throughout Italy and southern France.

Europe and Britain

In Northern Europe, however, society remained isolated and rural, based on a local agricultural economy. Physicians were available only to the higher ranks of society and the masses relied on folk healers. It is in this context that orthodox medicine arose in Britain. Three types of medicine, or healing, have been described as being practised in Britain in the 16th century, when orthodox medicine was beginning to emerge as a profession.[9]

The first was *official* (or orthodox) healing. This was endorsed by the newly established medical profession, taught in the universities, based upon physical knowledge available at that time and open to intellectual debate.

The second was *practical* healing, founded on folklore and involving the use of herbs and minerals. It may be worth considering that modern examples of practical healing could include the use of vitamins, arnica, cough remedies and herbal teas, none of which have established scientific support for their usefulness but have nevertheless achieved some respectability.

The third was *ritual* healing, consisting of the use of

charms, frequently derived from the prayers of the pre-Reformed church, witchcraft and sorcery.

Orthodox medicine was not always superior to the practical wisdom of the day. A striking illustration of this is the differing explanations given for outbreaks of syphilis which struck European ports in the late 15th century. Doctors of the prestigious University of Ferrara deemed that the disease resulted from a particular astrological event. Members of the Aberdeen Town Council pronounced that it was due to the presence in the town of sexually promiscuous women. It is always easy to be wise after the event!

From the beginning the Church was hostile to lay healing because of its presumed association with 'magic' and witchcraft. Misgivings about female practitioners were prevalent in the 16th century Church and lent further force to this opposition, with both witches and midwives being open to attack.

The first legal restriction of medical practice came in 1512 when an Act was passed which required the Church to supervise the competence of physicians. Six years later, concerned both to limit the unofficial practice of medicine and to establish national standards for orthodox medical practitioners, King Henry VIII founded the Royal College of Physicians in London. From this beginning orthodox medicine eventually emerged as having both political power and a monopoly over the explanation of disease and healing.

During the 15th and 16th centuries, expeditions to the American continents led to an international exchange of medical information. Quinine, a drug extracted from cinchona bark, was imported to Europe by explorers returning from Peru, where natives had for years used it to treat malaria. The realisation that quinine provided a precise solution to a particular set of symptoms paved the way for the introduction of other pharmacologically active compounds. Gradually new drugs were proposed, tried and accepted. Medical practice slowly changed from being a mixture of folklore and witchcraft to become a scientific discipline.

Progress in medicine in the 16th century in Britain was as influenced by European scientists outside the formal medical establishment as it is today. Politicians, engineers, physicists and chemists all played a role. Galileo developed the idea of a watch to measure the pulse rate, while one of his contemporaries, Sanctorius, designed and built the first weighing machine and clinical thermometer.

The microscope had a considerable impact on medical progress in the 17th century. Its development resulted from the work of several investigators in different countries. Robert Hooke, in London, was the first to use it to describe cells.

This equipment led to a new medical philosophy, expounded by men such as René Descartes, who regarded the human body as nothing more or less than a complex piece of machinery. Such an approach may have shocked the religious establishment but enabled rapid advances in medical science. The study of physiology began in earnest and provided the background on which future clinicians could develop diagnostic and therapeutic skills. William Harvey, who was the first scientist to prove that blood is pumped around the body in a closed circulatory system, is the best known British physiologist of this era.

All these developments contributed to the advancement of medical knowledge. The watch, thermometer, weighing machine and microscope enabled scientists to study the functioning of the human body with precision. Increased knowledge of basic physiology also followed Harvey's discovery. Old-fashioned theories were nevertheless slow to disappear.

One British 17th century physician who helped to prepare the medical profession for the new information provided by medical scientists was Thomas Sydenham. Basing his practice on that of Hippocrates, he was careful to make detailed observations of signs and symptoms. Sometimes refusing to use complex but ineffective remedies, he had a commonsense approach to therapy, prescribing iron for anaemia, quinine for malaria and opium for pain. This helped to establish within the British medical profession a new tradition of clinical observation and professional criticism.

In the 18th century, the Industrial Revolution, inspired by engineers and businessmen, dramatically altered living standards and disease patterns. Huge new factories and towns were built, and overcrowding and pollution were widespread. The new housing estates had no clean water supplies, no sewerage facilities and inadequate space for play or recreation.

The harmful effects on the British people did not become fully apparent for over a century, but one immediate result was an increase in the incidence of disease related to manufacturing processes. A number of physicians observed the new working conditions and made recommendations, such as masks for miners to protect their lungs and ventilation for workshops. Industrial medicine slowly developed into a speciality, although most of the recommendations were ignored as being too expensive.

Alcoholism, inevitably associated with child abuse and neglect, became prevalent as people tried to forget the miserable conditions in which they were working and living. The incidence of tuberculosis also rose, probably as a result of overcrowding, the damp cold climate and a window tax, which encouraged landlords to brick up their windows, thus depriving many people of air and light.

However, the 18th century also saw some breakthroughs. Edward Jenner, the son of a clergyman from Gloucestershire, revived the idea of vaccination against smallpox. Twenty years before a Dorset farmer, Benjamin Jesty, had vaccinated his wife and two sons with cowpox to protect them against smallpox. It had been observed that dairymaids who developed cowpox did not seem to get smallpox. The experiment was ignored by the medical profession. Edward Jenner repeated it and was successful, and news of his work spread around the world. During the next two hundred years, vaccination, first against smallpox and then against other diseases, was to prove the most effective weapon available to doctors for controlling infectious diseases.

The birth of the pharmaceutical industry owes much to the discovery by William Brockenden, born in Devon, that pills could be produced by reliable tablet-making machines, rather than being hand-rolled. This meant that doses of drugs could be standardised, and that pharmaceutical manufacturers could easily increase their profit by increasing their output. Later, apothecaries realised that it was easier and cheaper to buy their finished tablets from a specialist supplier.

Clinicians in the early 19th century started to put into practice the theoretical knowledge gained by medical scientists. René Laennec in France developed the stethoscope, and the microscope was used to study the pathology of specific disease processes. Thomas Addison, Thomas Hodgkin and James Parkinson were just three members of the British medical profession to give their names to specific diseases.

A long-established practice of selling corpses for dissection ultimately climaxed in scandal, and an Anatomy Act was passed in 1832 ruling that all unclaimed dead bodies should go to the medical schools for dissection. The study of anatomy was thus affirmed and became linked with clinical science.

The Industrial Revolution had by this time increased the number of people who could afford to buy professional medical care, and this led to an increased demand for properly recognised physicians and surgeons, rather than the services of unqualified quacks. The licensing and registration of physicians, surgeons and apothecaries thus became official.

While Jenner's vaccination was conquering smallpox, tuberculosis and cholera raged unchecked in the unhygienic living quarters of town inhabitants. In London alone the cholera outbreak of 1848–9 killed nearly 15,000 people. Edwin Chadwick, a civil servant, lawyer and journalist, studied the epidemiology of infectious diseases, using maps to show where the worst death rates occurred. He concluded and argued that proper sanitation would not only improve the quality of life but also be of economic value. His recommendations were incorporated into a Public Health Act in 1848, and were the driving force behind the development of clean water supplies and sewage disposal facilities.

Surgical mortality in the 19th century (despite the development of anaesthesia) was between 40 and 60%, with patients dying from infections although the surgery itself had been successful. Surgeons did not adopt any precautions against infection while operating. Louis Pasteur, a French chemist, developed the theory that fermentation is produced by small invisible organisms which could be destroyed by rapid heating.

Joseph Lister, a Scottish surgeon, read Pasteur's reports and realised the importance of keeping the hospital environment free of these small organisms which today we know as bacteria. He experimented with a variety of chemicals and eventually used carbolic acid as an antiseptic. It was another twenty years before his antiseptic techniques were widely adopted.

Following this, the work of Pasteur and a German doctor, Robert Koch, led to the development of vaccines against anthrax, rabies and cholera. Between them they founded the science of bacteriology, provided evidence for the mechanisms underlying the spread of infectious diseases, and showed that such diseases could be controlled.

In 1895 a fifty-year-old Professor of Physics at Würzburg in Germany made an accidental discovery which was to have as great an effect on modern medicine as any other technological innovation. Wilhelm Konrad von Röntgen accidentally discovered the existence of X-rays while studying the effects of cathode rays.

The efficiency of the printing industry had reached a peak. Röntgen published his work on 28 December 1895, and a month later the Lancet published an X-ray photograph of a human hand taken by a researcher in London. Radiography quickly became a speciality, and the value of X-rays in diagnosis was recognised worldwide.

By the early 20th century, medical science had developed so rapidly that no one person could be familiar with all the information and skills available to the clinician. Specialisation had become a necessity. For the first time, doctors began to call in colleagues for consultations. London was an obvious centre for specialists in Britain. Harley Street became a popular area to practise as it was conveniently close to two main-line railway stations, Euston and Paddington, and situated in a fashionable residential area.

Organised health services were gradually developed all over Europe. The first was introduced in Russia in 1862, followed by the scheme organised by the German government in 1880 and based partly on a programme of health insurance. This inspired the British Prime Minister Lloyd George to pass a National Health Insurance Act in 1911. This entitled wage-earners to sickness benefit and a free general practitioner service in return for regular contributions.

A rapid increase in the world population at the end of

the nineteenth century had dramatic effects on individual families. Whereas previously a woman could expect to lose half or more of her children in their first year of life, by the end of the century she could expect most of them to survive. Many people, supported by the rising feminist movement, began to demand birth-control. For many years only the simplest forms of contraceptives were available, and intra-uterine devices were only available to a very few women. Eventually oral contraceptives came on the market in the 1950s, and sterilisation became a simple and relatively painless operation.

By the early 20th century professional medical care was much more widely available. Patients could be protected from infections by vaccination, and accidental injuries could be dealt with surgically. Nevertheless, few effective drugs existed. Probably the most important were quinine, morphine, digitalis and aspirin. The first three had been available for several hundred years, and the fourth did not require a prescription.

The pharmacological revolution began in Germany, where Paul Ehrlich, a chemist, was searching for the 'magic bullet', a drug with specific activity against a specific disease. In 1910 he produced a substance called salvarsan which was an effective remedy for syphilis. Alexander Fleming's discovery of penicillin at St Mary's Hospital in London in 1928 was the result of good fortune as well as careful observation.

Antibiotics were the most important drugs to be added to the doctor's armoury in the 20th century. Before they were available, about 50% of patients who contracted pneumonia in the United States died. After the introduction of penicillin, mortality fell to approximately 5%.

There followed the introduction of the barbiturates, succeeded by other sedatives and tranquillisers. The science of endocrinology (the study of hormones) began at the start of the 20th century and led to the introduction of insulin to treat diabetes. Cortisone was isolated just after the Second World War and proved to be a vital tool in the treatment of various conditions including rheumatoid arthritis and asthma.

New vaccines were introduced against tetanus, diphtheria, tuberculosis and poliomyelitis. The importance of vitamin deficiencies and their correction were recognised. The World Health Organisation, established in 1946, enabled progress to be made in eradicating infectious diseases worldwide.

In 1948, the National Health Service was established in Britain. The provision of state support for the sick, elderly and disabled helped to eradicate poverty and minimise the economic consequences of illness. Nevertheless, such a service may have disadvantages for the doctor–patient relationship. These are discussed in chapter three.

Today it appears to some observers that medicine has lost some of its impetus. Medical care in Britain still concentrates on providing cures, rather than on prevention. An emphasis on prevention of heart disease, cancer and industrial hazards, to name just three, will be vital to the population's future health in developed countries.

In 1964, two scientists working in Cambridge, James Watson and Francis Crick, shared a Nobel Prize for elucidating the structure of deoxyribonucleic acid, or DNA. The discovery of the genetic code has introduced another field of study, that of molecular biology. Medical researchers are now confident that they can unravel the message of human inheritance. By the beginning of the 21st century they believe they will have located and analysed all the human genes on the DNA molecule and be able to load the entire set of instructions that specifies a human being into a computer database.

The Human Genome Project is the most ambitious scientific project since the Apollo project to land a man on the moon. We will have to wait to discover whether it will fulfil its hope of providing liberation from cancer, heart disease, auto-immune diseases such as rheumatoid arthritis and some psychiatric illnesses.

Conclusions

From this brief historical outline we can learn several lessons. Firstly, the distinction between orthodox and alternative medicine is to some extent an artificial one, although there may be excellent reasons for making that distinction.

Secondly, religion and medicine have always been associated. The church has for a number of reasons allied itself with orthodox medicine in the past, and the intellectual and religious debates over the validity of alternative medicine did not originate in the twentieth century.

Thirdly, throughout history the sick have had recourse to practitioners of orthodox medicine as well as to spiritual leaders and 'folk medicine'. We can therefore distinguish between two types of alternative medicine: those which are based on sometimes harmless and useful folklore, and those which have a definite spiritual, or religious significance. As we shall see later, some forms of alternative therapy practised today may be regarded as belonging to either one or to both groups, depending on one's viewpoint.

While from an economic and scientific perspective it may be important to try to eliminate ineffective therapies based on folklore alone, I do not believe that it is about these therapies that Christians are most concerned. Rather, those therapies with a specific spiritual significance are those which are most worrying. There are many reasons why, in a supposedly 'scientific' age, such therapies are becoming more widely established, and these will be considered in the next chapter.

Fourthly, modern medicine owes much to contributions

from non-medical scientists. The beneficial role of research and the importance of interaction between clinicians and non-clinical scientists must not be underestimated in the future.

Finally, orthodox medicine is not always correct in its interpretation of established scientific knowledge. It follows that orthodox medicine may later be shown to have been incorrect in its deductions. Opinions based upon practical knowledge cannot always be lightly dismissed. Christians should realise that orthodox medicine does not always have all the answers. The medical profession needs to be honest enough to admit this when appropriate and continue to widen its horizons of knowledge.

3

WHY ALTERNATIVE MEDICINE?

Cured yesterday of my disease, I died last night of my physician.

Matthew Prior in *The Remedy Worse than the Disease*

News about him [Jesus] spread . . . people brought to him all who were ill with various diseases, those suffering severe pain, the demon-possessed, those having seizures, and the paralysed, and he healed them.

Matthew 4:24

In this chapter I want to explore some of the reasons for the recent surge of interest in alternative medicine. In order to assess intelligently what our response to alternative medicine should be, it is not enough merely to note the statistics quoted previously. We should also have some idea of what makes it so attractive.

Medical Progress

Greater Hope

The advent of modern medicine, including surgery and anaesthetics, has dramatically altered the outcome for a number of medical and surgical conditions. This is particularly true for acute illness resulting from infectious diseases. We often forget that Alexander Fleming only discovered penicillin a little over sixty years ago, in

1928. Until this time there was no specific remedy for such a common illness as pneumonia, which was frequently fatal. Childhood infections such as rheumatic fever and whooping cough also claimed many casualties. Numerous women died in childbirth and infant mortality was high. Tuberculosis was a frequent cause of death, not sparing the famous, such as the fictional heroine of Verdi's 'La Traviata', composed in 1853, or the British writer George Orwell in this century.

The following figures illustrate some of these changes.[1] Life expectancy at birth in 1840 in England and Wales was forty years; by 1989 it had risen to seventy-three years for men and seventy-eight years for women. Infant deaths in the UK in 1870 were 150 per 1000 live births; by 1990 they had fallen to 8 per 1000. In 1950 only 3.5% of the UK population was aged 75 and over; by 1990 that figure had almost doubled to 6.7%.

Today we have to go to famine or war-stricken countries to see disease claim so many lives on such a widespread scale. Alternatively we can gain glimpses of what life in Europe was like from reading contemporary accounts, such as Thomas Mann's description of a tuberculosis sanatorium.[2] Lewis Thomas gives us some idea of the revolution in medicine in North America afforded by new technology developed in the 1920s and the resulting changes which affected patients and doctors alike.[3]

The 'miracles' of modern medicine are apparently now largely taken for granted. Patients often assume the availability of 'high-tech' treatments. A middle-aged man with newly-diagnosed angina may discuss the possibility of cardiac transplantation in much the same way as he discusses his anti-anginal tablets. Even a patient with lung cancer may assume that chemotherapy offers long-term, disease-free survival. These patients are understandably very frightened, so they will naturally search for the most effective treatment, but it is noteworthy that their expectations, quite alien from those of even our grand-parents, have been raised.

Where do these expectations come from? To some extent the medical profession itself has been responsible for creating them. In our enthusiasm over all that modern medicine has to offer, and in our desire to ensure that no-one will miss out, we have boldly and confidently publicised our achievements. In the last twenty years, quick to take advantage of a new story, journalists have seized on every new development. The results of successes (and recently, failures) have been published in newspapers and on television. In this country and abroad it is now commonplace for the latest studies reported in the BMJ, Lancet or other international medical journals to be discussed on radio and television programmes. The public is better informed than ever before and hopes for consistent results from the medical profession.

Greater Disappointment

Our well-informed public, with high anticipations of all that modern medicine can offer, is particularly susceptible to disappointment. There are two major causes of disenchantment: chronic disease and drug toxicity.

The Treatment That Doesn't Exist

Chronic disease is an obvious source of disappointment. Despite great achievements in this century, especially in treating infectious diseases, conventional medicine still has few effective remedies for many recurrent illnesses. There are numerous examples. In most cases we are unable to offer cures for quite common conditions such as asthma, recurrent back pain, epilepsy, diabetes and migraine, to name but a few.

Where striking advances have been made, such as the use of kidney transplants to treat chronic renal failure, complications such as organ rejection may still arise and recovery be incomplete. The economic resources may not always be available for transplantation, and even if they are, a suitable donor may not be found.

The problem of ineffective treatment for chronic disease has been compounded in the past by the generally recognised (although often ignored) truth that acute health care problems are generally regarded as being more prestigious. They have therefore often attracted more ambitious physicians and greater government resources (for example funding for research) than areas of chronic illness.

The present British government's recent emphasis on achieving certain health targets (for example improved care of patients with asthma) could potentially improve this situation. However, long-term changes will require increased funding as well as goodwill, or research into prevention and better treatments will cease and new doctors will not be attracted into these fields.

The Treatment That Does Exist

Another cause of disappointment is the treatment patients *do* receive. With the widespread use of potent drugs with potentially dangerous side-effects, patients are becoming increasingly aware of their possible dangers. Alternative therapies may therefore appear attractive because they are promoted as offering 'natural' and supposedly safe remedies. As we shall see later, this is often a fallacy, and one which should be exposed to public scrutiny.

My Doctor Seems Remote

When infections such as bubonic plague, typhus, tuberculosis and syphilis were usually lethal despite all the doctor's efforts, the doctor often had nothing to offer the patient for palliation, let alone cure. Consequently physicians learnt to give a sympathetic word and a handshake to victims sometimes shunned by friends or relatives. Physical contact was undoubtedly important in imparting confidence to patients, and was developed to a fine art in the techniques of organ palpation and the use of the stethoscope. Even today a patient coming for a routine out-patient appointment may ask for the reassurance of a physical examination.

Very often the doctor was present at the patient's death, providing some comfort to both the patient and the family. Thus the doctor performed a role as a trusted friend, usually alongside the local religious leader, or priest in Christian countries.

Today modern technology has rendered such contact impracticable. Patients are often treated in hospital, in unfamiliar and clinical surroundings. Those in the coronary care unit following a heart attack (a universally frightening experience) are conscious of flickering and alarming monitors. Those with terminal cancer for whom 'nothing can be done' are often shunned by the busy house officer, for whom such contact is both uncomfortable and time-consuming. If patients do not feel understood and cared for, they may look for alternative sources of support.

As alluded to in chapter three, the structure and organisation of the National Health Service itself may also be partly to blame. The percentage of hospital employees directly involved in patient care has fallen since its inception, while the percentage of administrative staff has risen dramatically. New hospitals therefore tend to be designed along patterns which meet the requirements of administrators rather than those of patients.

In a 12th century hospital the patients' ward was the most important part of the building, whereas in a modern centre of excellence, for whatever good reasons, wards occupy only about 20% of the space. Hospitals are usually built as multi-storey blocks, rather than along the lines recommended by Florence Nightingale, even though modern evidence supports the view that her favoured pavilion approach is better for patients.

Long waiting lists, industrial action by ancillary staff and the absence of casualty departments in some hospitals have contributed to the deterioration in the doctor–patient relationship. In the entire history of medicine there has probably never before been a time when a patient was turned away from a hosptial.

My Doctor Is Too Busy

In general practice, consultations may take seven minutes or less. Few worries or confidences can be shared in such a short time, even though the doctor can make an accurate diagnosis. There are tests, maybe pills, maybe a smile and a handshake, but rarely anything more. There may be no time to listen, and this is frustrating for many doctors as well as for the patient. The doctor has lost the role of trusted friend and has become a technical expert.

Where general practitioners have tried to increase their consultation times, patients may then feel daunted by the consulting room computer which has been introduced as a time-saving measure. It can be disconcerting for the patient to talk to a doctor who spends four of those seven minutes peering at a computer screen, thereby reducing even eye contact almost to zero.

The same problem has arisen in hospitals. With more advanced technology available, doctors are busier than ever before. The cardiac arrest bleep has replaced the night porter in alerting the duty physician to a patient's collapse and imminent death. Such a call therefore entails several hours' work in resuscitating the patient and, if successful, transferring him or her to the intensive care unit.

During the day, the electronic bleep is a constant source of disruption for junior doctors. The calls sometimes appear trivial, perhaps because the nurse on duty is inexperienced, and the constant interruptions make even routine tasks frustratingly difficult.

Increasing 'day surgery' means that some patients spend under twenty-four hours in hospital. The house officer may face a formidable task as he or she tries to clerk the patients in time for theatre, even when necessary investigations are completed during a prior clinic visit. The consultant surgeon has less time to talk to the patient and listen to his or her concerns.

Hospital consultants are also busier in other areas. They often have increased roles in administration and the responsibility for organising hospital audit. They may be required to comply with goals and standards set by hospital managers, for example to reduce outpatient waiting times. Such goals are excellent and very desirable, as anyone who has waited in an outpatients department knows well, but unless there are adequate numbers of doctors to perform the clinics, they may be unrealistic.

Whether doctors continue to enjoy such challenges or whether they leave the profession is irrelevant to this discussion. What is clear is that it is difficult for the most caring and conscientious doctor working in such situations to devote very much time to a patient's worries. An anxious and frightened patient may understandably feel let down.

Shifts In Disease Patterns

As noted previously there has been a striking decline in the death rate in Britain since the advent of industrialisation. This is owing to reductions in childhood and infectious diseases largely resulting from better water supplies, drainage and facilities for refuse disposal. Obviously if people do not die in childhood or early adult life they must die of something else later in life. There have been significant rises in the proportion of deaths due to cancer, circulatory disease (heart attacks and strokes), drug addiction, accidents and violent crime. The following figures illustrate some of this trend. In 1961 circulatory disease accounted for approximately 40% of deaths in men aged 60; in 1982 it accounted for 55% of deaths in the same group. In 1961 cancer caused 30% of deaths in women aged 60; in 1982 it was responsible for over 40% of deaths in the same group.[4] Cancer is therefore claiming lives which might otherwise have been lost to diphtheria, rheumatic fever or tuberculosis.

So far, modern medicine has been relatively ineffective in the face of these new 'epidemics', and this throws into stark relief the greater expectations of patients.

Social Progress

Single Households

Since the 1960s there has been a significant increase in the proportion of households containing people living alone and single parents with dependent children.[5] Several factors have contributed to this.

Firstly, increased life-expectancy, itself the product of modern medicine, means that a greater proportion of households contain only one elderly person. Secondly, increased mobility has led to a greater number of people leaving their home and town or village to live and work amongst strangers. Thirdly, changes in society's moral values have resulted in an increase in the number of households containing unmarried or divorced people. This often means that contact with family or friends is reduced, and those living alone may not find support in times of illness quite so readily. Some may turn instead to their general practitioner for support. If a sympathetic ear and time for listening are not forthcoming, they may more readily turn to an alternative therapist.

Rejection of Religion

Between 1970 and 1985, recorded membership of Christian churches in the UK fell from 20% of the adult population to 15%.[6] These membership figures tend to overestimate church attendance because they include those whose membership has lapsed. It is estimated that only one in ten people in Britain attends church regularly today. Non-churchgoers today are extremely unlikely to have any kind or relationship with their local vicar or with lay members of the church, who previously could have been a source of comfort in times of illness.

In a society where belief in medicine has largely replaced a belief in God, many doctors are failing to fulfil the role previously played by church ministers. People no longer trust a God they do not believe in with the outcome of their illness, and many are desperate. Those whom modern medicine can neither cure nor comfort will turn just about anywhere else in their quest for help and encouragement.

A Multicultural Society

Immigration is not a new phenomenon in Britain.[7] It has been estimated that in the 18th century there were 20,000 black people living in this country, and in the 19th century large numbers of Irish immigrants entered England, particularly during the potato famines in the 1840s.

Nevertheless, after the Second World War, immigration from the Commonwealth, particularly from the Caribbean, was actively encouraged in order to meet labour shortages during the 1950s. At present over 80% of West Indian teenagers were born in Britain, showing that these immigrants have settled in this country and had families. Asians, Indians and Pakistanis form the bulk of other ethnic minorities.

Without doubt we now live in a multi-racial society.

This can contribute to the increasing demand for alternative therapies in several ways. Immigrants recently arrived from developing countries may have different expectations of doctors and medicine. They will probably expect time and contact with the physician and may be less familiar with modern technology.

They may collectively bring alternative remedies with them. A particularly striking example of this is seen in the widespread market for Chinese remedies, particularly for eczema, which are sold in London's Chinatown.

The first generation of settlers at least is more likely to belong to the poorer sections of the community. This group will thereby be subject to the inequalities in health outlined below.

The Gap Between Rich and Poor

In many societies, the lower down the social scale individuals find themselves, the less healthy they are and the shorter their life expectancy. The reasons will differ between countries but the following examples illustrate some of them.

Where medical care has to be paid for directly by the patient to the doctor or hospital, those who are poorer will tend to avoid seeking medical help if at all possible. This will often mean that problems thought by the patient and his or her family to be less serious will be neglected. In addition, where receiving medical care involves travelling some distance, for instance to a specialised hospital, those on lower incomes may not feel able to continue receiving such treatment because of the prohibitive cost of public transport.

Certain occupations have health risks associated with them. Obvious examples are asbestos and coal mining. Traditionally these are occupations taken up by the poorer members of society, who then become more likely to develop lung disease.

Families on poorer incomes in any country tend to have restricted access to the best education provided by that country. The cumulative result of generations of poor education is a diminished understanding of the causes of disease and measures for prevention.

Finally, low income has a direct adverse effect on diet and therefore nutrition. A lowered consumption of fresh meat, fish, vegetables and fruit, which in western countries tend to be more expensive than so-called 'junk foods' high in fat and sugar, may have adverse consequences on a person's health.

When the NHS was founded in 1948, it was established that medical care in Britain should be paid for by indirect taxation and that all should have access to medical care regardless of income. Nevertheless, the gap between the health of the poor and the rich remains in Britain today. It was highlighted by the Report of the Working Group on Inequalities in Health (known as the Black Report) in 1980 and has been confirmed by independent reports since then. Notable exemptions from the principle of free medical care are prescription charges and the fees charged by dentists and opticians.

Of greater concern, however, is that differences in mortality (death rates) and morbidity (sickness rates) between the rich and the poor have continued to increase since 1980. As chronic diseases now constitute a greater proportion of all diseases in the UK, the relationship between mortality and morbidity is weaker than previously. Therefore studying death rates alone may not yield a true reflection of health in this country today. The NHS is thus failing to ensure equality of medical care throughout society and many are consequently disillusioned with conventional medicine.

A further inequality in society is the use of the health service by men and women. Women are the biggest users of health care facilities, reflecting their responsibilities as child-bearers and child-rearers. The feminists have taken up this issue and 'well-women clinics' are an attempt to address it. However, women remain at present poorly represented among the higher ranks of the medical profession. Some women may therefore seek to control their own medical care by turning to alternative practitioners who may not carry such a patriarchal or paternalistic image.

What Does Alternative Medicine Offer?

Time

Alternative practitioners offer time. They offer time to listen to patients and time to explain their problem to them. An average first session with an alternative practitioner lasts one hour, at least twice that generally afforded for a first consultation with a hospital consultant. Time invested by a practitioner communicates care and compassion to the patient. It may also give the patient a sense of greater control over his or her future.

Touch

The traditional handshake, the ritual pulse-taking and the arm around the shoulder, seem rather old-fashioned now and may be disappearing. Doctors are probably afraid of appearing condescending and medical students are increasingly taught that the patient should be a partner in his or her treatment.

One unforeseen consequence of this teaching is that patients are increasingly being offered a selection of treatments and then being advised to make the choice themselves. Although this approach may be appropriate for some, others may find it unnerving. When people feel unwell and vulnerable, they can find it particularly difficult to make important decisions with far-reaching consequences. Such an attitude on the part of the doctor may also imply that none of the treatments on offer are particularly effective, so that it doesn't really matter which one the patient receives. This also is unhelpful, as we shall see later when discussing the 'placebo' effect.

Without exerting any specific effect on the disease, touch expresses involvement and can make people 'feel better'. In the long run this is what most patients want. Many alternative therapies provide a degree of physical contact and thereby reassurance not afforded by conventional medicine. Various forms of massage, and aromatherapy, are examples of alternative therapies which provide substantial physical contact with the patient.

Trust

It is well known that the 'gut feeling' of either the doctor or the patient about a particular treatment is not always a good guide to how effective that treatment really is. This is partly because both doctors and patients tend to be biased in favour of treatment, and partly because of the placebo phenomenon.

'Placebo' literally means, 'I shall please'. Originally a placebo was a pharmacologically inert compound prepared to satisfy the patient's desire for treatment rather than specifically to treat his or her disease. Some placebos might have pharmacological activity not specifically effective for the illness, an example being a vitamin preparation given as a 'tonic' to a patient who is not vitamin-deficient.

One third of all people given an inert compound to relieve a particular symptom will report relief of that symptom.[8] This phenomenon is known as the 'placebo effect'. The placebo response can be altered by the style of the presentation of the drug or its route of administration (such as tablets or injections). For example, one study has shown that red placebo tablets were more effective in relieving pain than were blue ones, and these in turn were more effective than green ones.[9]

The confidence of both the doctor and the patient in a particular drug can profoundly affect the patient's response to treatment. Much early medicine consisted of rituals which were effective to some extent if the patient believed in them. The patient's trust in the practitioner's ability to heal also augments the placebo response.

Current technology in medicine is removing the placebo effect in medicine. Computers, scanners and biochemical analyzers can provide diagnostic tests and be used to deliver and control therapy. If doctors have insufficient time to impart confidence, the only area where the placebo effect will still play a role is in the colour, shape and size of tablets.

Alternative medicine, by providing the patient with new and sometimes rather exotic explanations and treatments, restores some of the mystery of medicine and may reinforce belief in the practitioner's skills. Where conventional medicine has failed, an alternative practitioner's confident arguments for the cause and remedy of the disease may sound very convincing.

Sometimes it Really Works

In some cases, alternative medicine does offer an effective treatment. Until recently, osteopathy was regarded by the medical profession as potentially hazardous and probably ineffective. Now it is increasingly offered by general practitioners alongside conventional medicine. Some studies have shown that patients derive greater benefit from osteopathy than from other forms of treatment, particularly for chronic low back pain, and the Osteopaths Act passed in 1993 provides for regulation of all osteopathic practitioners. Osteopathy is set to become part of future mainstream medicine.

A Spiritual Dimension

The decline in interest in mainstream religion and Christianity in this country does not necessarily mean that people don't want spiritual support in times of illness. It merely means that many have turned to other sources. We have already noted the link between disease and spiritual beliefs. Now that medicine no longer offers answers as to the significance of the illness or the threat of death, some alternative therapies may offer a spiritual dimension not found in the NHS.

It is precisely because some alternative therapies *do* work that they can all be attractive to the desperate patient. They are also relatively difficult to evaluate scientifically, making it difficult to distinguish fact from fiction. How we might begin to do this is the subject of the next chapter.

Controversy is Not New

Before proceeding to the next chapter, I should like to emphasise something which may be useful to recall when considering these controversial issues. Dissatisfaction with the medical profession is not new; doctors have always had to contend with criticism and complaints. In the light of the factors outlined above it is therefore perhaps not surprising that doctors today are increasingly unable to meet their patients' expectations, despite the dramatic therapeutic progress made in some fields.

Part II

4

ALTERNATIVE MEDICINE: THE PROBLEMS

The wisdom of the prudent is to give thought to their ways.
Proverbs 14:8

There are two equal and opposite errors into which our race can fall about the devils. One is to disbelieve in their existence. The other is to believe, and to feel an excessive and unhealthy interest in them. They themselves are equally pleased by both errors.

C.S. Lewis *The Screwtape Letters*

In this chapter I want to look at some of the evidence for there being genuine risks associated with the various practices of alternative medicine. This is necessary before deciding how best to approach them.

At this point I shall attempt to classify the main types of alternative therapy currently practised. There is no unifying concept underlying them; they are merely grouped together because they lie outside the scope of conventional medicine. Their diversity of approach means that they are not easily amenable to classification, and are frequently listed alphabetically. Nevertheless, I believe that, however crude a classification may be, it helps to understand both the rationale and potential hazards associated with each one. For definitions of individual therapies the reader is referred to chapter seven.

I have grouped therapies according to their method of

delivery, that is, external (physical), internal or psychic. Some treatments encompass more than one of these, but I find the distinction nevertheless helpful.

External (Physical) Treatments

These involve massage or manipulation.

Examples: Acupuncture, the Alexander technique, aromatherapy, chiropractic, osteopathy, kinesiology, reflexology and shiatsu.

Internal Treatments

These involve taking medicines (sometimes rather attractively called elixirs, oils or infusions) internally (usually by mouth, although I would include enemas in this section).

Examples: Bach flower remedies, herbalism and homoeopathy.

Psychic Treatments

These are therapies which are either psychological in origin or paranormal, the latter making use of forces not recognised by natural laws.

Examples: Crystal therapy, hypnotherapy, radionics and transcendental meditation.

A noticeable feature of many alternative therapies is that as a group they make considerable use of physical and psychic treatments. In contrast, orthodox medicine relies on taking medicine or performing surgical procedures. This has implications for the types of hazards which can result from alternative medicine.

The Risks of Alternative Medicine

According to the main emphasis of any particular remedy, potential hazards can also be classified as being physical, directly affecting physical functioning of one or more organs in the body, or psychic, when the effects may involve more subtle effects on people's mental state, beliefs or psychological experiences.

Physical Hazards

One of the most misleading statements often made about herbal remedies is that because they are 'natural' they cannot cause harm. The following examples frankly contradict this claim.

Herbal Remedies

There are now reported to be over 600 clinics offering traditional Chinese medicine in the United Kingdom.[1] Chinese herbal remedies are especially well-known for their success in eczema. Eczema is a distressing skin condition frequently affecting children. It can cause misery through constant itching, sleepless nights and skin disfigurement resulting in social isolation. Chinese herbal remedies have produced dramatic improvement in some patients in whom the condition had previously been resistant to orthodox treatment. Parents are therefore understandably under considerable pressure to try such treatments when conventional medicine has failed to bring relief.

However, there is increasing concern about the safety of these remedies. There is accumulating evidence that they may contain both uncharacterised compounds with serious and poorly documented side-effects, and potent conventional pharmacological agents with well-known hazards.

There are a number of reports in the medical literature of liver toxicity, in at least one case fatal, associated with Chinese herbal remedies.[2] Such hazards may affect Chinese patients in China, or British patients taking these treatments in this country.

Combined liver and kidney failure (hepatorenal failure)

has also been attributed to the toxic effects of a herbal medicine taken by a Chinese man.[3] Analysis of its ingredients showed that it contained, amongst others, benzaldehyde, cinnamoyl alcohol, ephedrine, orange peel and pigeon droppings. To take just one of these as an example, ephedrine, used in some 'over the counter' formulations as a nasal decongestant, stimulates the release of an adrenaline-like compound and can cause rises in heart rate and blood pressure. This is potentially dangerous in patients with heart disease, high blood pressure or an overactive thyroid, and presents risks for patients taking a particular type of antidepressants known as monoamine oxidase inhibitors. The toxicity of pigeon droppings can only be guessed at. Kidney failure of sudden onset was reported in six patients seen at the Kenyatta National Hospital, two of whom died.[4] All became ill within ten to seventy hours of taking herbal folk remedies which were claimed to treat infertility and abdominal pain.

In March 1992 a traditional healer was sentenced in London to three years in prison for giving patients near fatal doses of mercury and arsenic.[5] A review of deaths in the Transvaal thought to be due to herbal remedies found that the main toxic ingredient was digitalis.[6] Digitalis, originally derived from the foxglove, is used in orthodox medicine to treat certain heart disorders. However, it is always used judiciously because of its well-documented toxicity, and many doctors monitor blood levels at some stage during treatment.

In Thailand, traditional anti-malarial remedies sold in rural groceries have been found to contain antihistamines, steroids, vitamins, antibiotics and pain-killers in addition to orthodox antimalarial agents such as quinine or pyrimethamine.[7]

There are also reports of Chinese herbal remedies containing potent steroids. This seems particularly ironic at a time when more patients (and their parents) than ever before are questioning the safety of steroids prescribed by orthodox medical practitioners for a variety of conditions, and may turn to 'natural' herbal treatments as a safer alternative. A Chinese herbal remedy purchased in Manchester for treatment of a boy's facial eczema was found to contain fluocinolone, which is a potent steroid. This is particularly worrying since the application of potent steroids to the face can result in thinning of the skin, permanent scarring and severe dermatitis.

A fifty-four year old woman was investigated at the Victoria Infirmary, Glasgow, for postmenopausal bleeding.[8] Results of tests suggested that hormonal stimulation was the cause. Prior to this she had also consulted a homoeopath about perimenopausal symptoms. He had prescribed her a remedy called APITOP-F. The accompanying leaflet stated that this agent was a 'vitamin-hormone' which would treat numerous conditions including menstrual irregularities. The ingredients included ethinyloestradiol, an oestrogen which may be prescribed to women on a short-term basis only for perimenopausal symptoms. No warnings were given in the leaflet and it was stated that the preparation could be given long-term. The use of oestrogens in women during and after the menopause is associated with an increased risk of developing cancer of the womb.

Aconite poisoning from Chinese herbal remedies has also been reported.[9] In China over 600 cases have been reported in the last thirty years and the problem is thought to be widespread in Chinese communities worldwide.

The problem is not confined to Chinese herbal remedies. Liver damage developed in four women who took so-called natural remedies, 'Kalms' and 'Neurelax', to relieve stress.[10] It is thought that the poisonous substances were valerian (a sedative drug from the dried roots of valerian) and skullcap, a perennial flowering plant. Kalms and Neurelax are sold in health food shops and recommended for the relief of stress. They are promoted as non-habit forming, natural plant remedies without side-effects. On a lighter note, valerian and skullcap are also among the ingredients of certain 'natural' remedies recommended for 'nervous conditions' in cats, including travel sickness.

There are problems in India too. A three-month-old baby died after being given a traditional Indian medicine for constipation.[11] Post-mortem examination revealed peritonitis and a severely damaged stomach lining. An Indian eye remedy called surma, containing up to 86% lead, has been responsible for causing lead poisoning in a number of children.

A so-called homoeopathic herbal remedy from India for the treatment of asthma was found to contain a steroid.[12] This ingredient would explain its effectiveness, but steroids also have potentially hazardous side-effects. In the course of normal medical practice, these are usually minimised by careful prescribing and monitoring. However, if the patient and medical practitioner are unaware that the patient is receiving steroids, such side-effects may develop and go both unrecognised and untreated.

These examples illustrate at least four problems associated with such remedies.

1. Ingredients are unknown At present, the ingredients in most alternative remedies do not have to be declared, so both patients and doctors may be unaware of their contents.

2. Ingredients may be toxic Such treatments may contain drugs used in conventional medicine which are known to have potentially dangerous side-effects. The doses may exceed those which would usually be prescribed by orthodox practitioners.

3. Contamination may exist   Since there is currently no legal requirement for tests of purity and content, there may be unrecognised contamination with undesirable substances. These may include other herbs, drugs, and various chemicals (for example heavy metals and insecticides) as well as even less desirable items.

4. Ingredients may interact   Finally, the active ingredients present in these formulations may interact with orthodox medicines already prescribed for the patient by a medical doctor. Such interactions may have grave consequences.

As a result of these concerns, the National Poisons Unit at Guy's Hospital in London now collects information on cases where the use of alternative remedies has led to patients becoming ill. Since 1985 hundreds of enquiries have been made about poisoning with herbal medicines.

Are the Risks Greater than for Orthodox Medicine?

It may be argued that many alternative medicines have been used for centuries with few ill effects. The cases given above may represent only exceptional incidents used to increase prejudice within the medical profession against such remedies. Since orthodox medicines can be so toxic, why are doctors so concerned about occasional side-effects resulting from the use of herbal remedies?

There are several reasons for serious concern. Side-effects resulting from these remedies are unpredictable. This is because the ingredients are usually not listed on the packaging. Even if they are listed there may be little medical experience of such agents or of their interaction with orthodox remedies. Furthermore, there may be unintentional contamination with other harmful substances.

Since side-effects are unpredictable, patients cannot be

forewarned about them. It again seems ironic that, in the search for greater patient freedom, patients have in fact taken giant leaps backwards, not forwards. While insisting that they are better informed with regard to the hazards of modern drugs and surgery, they are risking serious poisoning from substances about which they have either little or no information whatsoever.

As discussed in the next chapter, much of the information that is given with alternative remedies is misleading and some of it is frankly untrue. Some Christians may go further and view the lies as a direct result of evil, but whatever one's interpretation it is clearly irresponsible to allow this situation to persist.

Natural Does Not Mean Harmless

I am particularly concerned that patients often believe the claim that these remedies are 'natural' and therefore harmless, even if they prove to be ineffective. In the face of inadequate or unpleasant orthodox therapy, the temptation to try them then becomes almost irresistible. The above examples show that 'natural' or herbal remedies can be extremely toxic. Conversely, a significant number of powerful modern drugs have been developed from herbal sources. However, this in no way means that they are harmless, as the following examples illustrate.

Curare is a resin obtained from certain tropical trees. Owing to its ability to cause muscular paralysis and death in sufficient doses it was used by the South American Indians as an arrow poison. Nevertheless, derivatives of curare, such as tubocurarine and pancuronium, are now routinely administered during surgical anaesthesia to induce muscle relaxation.

Digitalis was originally isolated from the pretty foxglove of rural England. In 1776 William Withering, a Birmingham physician, described its effectiveness in the treatment of dropsy or ankle swelling, now known to be a feature of some forms of heart disease. He himself had learnt about the usefulness of foxglove leaves from an elderly lady he had met while travelling to Shropshire. Today, digitalis remains an important weapon in the treatment of heart disease. It is given to treat irregularities of heart rhythm and to improve the pumping action of the heart. Despite its natural origin, digitalis can be hazardous and its use requires careful monitoring. It can cause fatal irregularities of the heartbeat rhythm at relatively low circulating concentrations. Less severe side-effects include loss of appetite, nausea, vomiting, diarrhoea, confusion, psychiatric disturbances and visual disturbances including photophobia, blurring of vision and disordered colour vision.

Aspirin is derived from a compound isolated from the graceful willow tree. Its value was highlighted in 1763 by a paper to the Royal Society of Medicine entitled 'An account of the success of the bark of the willow in the cure of the agues'. Its scientific name, salicylate, comes from the Latin name for willow (*salix*). Aspirin has pain-relieving and anti-inflammatory properties and effectively reduces fever. Even in normal doses it causes a small degree of gastro-intestinal bleeding. In prolonged therapy, or in patients with a predisposition to gastro-intestinal bleeding, it may cause life-threatening blood loss. In cases of self-poisoning with aspirin, the subject may develop tinnitus (ringing in the ears), deafness, a high fever with sweating and dehydration, stomach pains, vomiting, gastro-intestinal haemorrhage, reduced blood sugar levels, respiratory disturbances and impaired consciousness.

Morphine, a powerful pain-killer, was isolated from the South West Asian poppy (*Papaver somniferum*), an attractive plant with greyish-green leaves and white or reddish flowers. Morphine relieves severe pain and is widely used in pre-operative medication. It may be used in heart disease and helps suppress coughing. However, the sedative and euphoric effects of morphine and related compounds have led to long-standing worldwide abuse, exemplified in England by opium dens in the 19th century and intravenous heroin addiction in the 20th century. Less alluring side effects include respiratory depression, nausea, vomiting and constipation.

Atropine is a modern drug derived from the deadly nightshade (*Atropa belladonna*). It has a variety of uses which include reduction of secretions prior to surgery, treatment of the very slow pulse which can follow a heart attack, dilating pupils prior to eye examination, relief of airway narrowing in asthma, treatment of Parkinson's disease and prevention of travel sickness. Side-effects include drying of the mouth, blurred vision, constipation, glaucoma in susceptible individuals, confusion, restlessness and hallucinations.

I hope I have now convinced the reader that 'natural' remedies are by no means harmless just because they are isolated from natural sources such as plants. There is no such thing as a 'good' drug or a 'bad' drug. All of the drugs discussed above are extremely valuable tools in medicine and yet may be fatal in overdose. This fallacy is one which all professionals involved in patient education should firmly destroy once and for all.

Psychic Risks

It is obviously difficult to define such risks. However, it does appear that there are effects associated with certain types of alternative therapies, often those where psychic treatments are involved, which are not physical in nature. It is even more difficult to be precise about the extent and nature of such effects. Given that most medical practitioners and much of the public question the existence of the paranormal realm altogether, this is not surprising.

Much evidence is anecdotal and coloured by personal prejudices and beliefs. Nevertheless, as outlined above, many alternative therapies do have their origins in the psychic realm and I will now examine just a few of these.

Some Obvious Problems

A popular concept in many branches of alternative medicine is that of a 'life force' or 'vital energy' within the body. Christians should be aware that the theme of 'energy' is also the unifying thread which runs through the diverse dogmas of the New Age movement. Following directly from ancient Chinese beliefs, good health is sometimes said to depend upon a balance between its two components, referred to as 'yin' and 'yang'.

Two alternative therapies developed from such beliefs include yoga and transcendental meditation (TM). They are based on Hindu religious philosophy. The purpose of yoga, as taught by Hindu teachers, is to unite the human spirit with Hindu gods by means of various physical postures. Hindu teachers of yoga believe that all yoga is a religious exercise, that each position represents an act of worship to a Hindu god and that the physical exercises cannot be divorced from spiritual involvement.

For Christians, therefore, it seems clear that the practice of yoga or TM are not valid options since we are to worship the one and only living God. For non-Christians there is a choice, but it would be reasonable for all doctors and patients to be made aware that these are not strictly medical, but religious practices.

Other terms for these 'energies' include naturopathy's 'vital force', Mesmer's 'magnetism', 'cosmic energy', 'universal energy', 'chi life force' and 'biomagnetic'. Many practitioners believe that healing energy can be transmitted directly from one person to another.

The not so Obvious Problems

It is not always clear when alternative therapies involve psychic practices. Terms for healing are often used which may sound quite rational, or at least harmless and acceptable to Christians. These include 'massage', 'laying on of hands', 'holistic' and 'wellness'.

Jane Gumprecht[13] emphasises an association between healing promoted by the New Age movement and many alternative therapies practised in the USA. As a Christian doctor whose parents were enticed into New Age philosophies, she is well qualified to discuss the subject. Some examples of her conclusions are given below.

Dr Gumprecht attributes the overwhelming American emphasis on strenuous exercise to New Age influence. She points out that excessive exercise can be hazardous, resulting in sudden death, musculo-skeletal injuries and infertility in young women. Medical studies show only a modest effect of moderate exercise on heart disease and do not support a beneficial effect for strenuous exercise. It is well known that strenuous exercise leads to euphoria or a 'natural high'. Jane Gumprecht believes that the New Age goal is to promote heightened awareness.

One does not necessarily have to accept this view of New Age involvement in order to perceive the nature of the attraction. What makes people devote excessive time and money to strenuous exercise? I suspect it is a morbid fear of illness, a desire to be fashionable, or both. Such motives are evident.

The Bible teaches that it is right to take care of our physical bodies.[14] When afraid of illness it is appropriate to examine our lifestyles to see if anything should be altered. We would be well advised to seek medical advice when concerned. A brisk daily walk, balanced diet, reduction in alcohol intake and cessation of smoking are all prudent precautions.

However, part of the Bible's teaching is that mankind tends to worship what is created (for example, animals or birds, the sun and the stars, money or material possessions) rather than the one God who created these things.[15] Such created things, when they become more important to us than God, are described as idols.

If as Christians we pursue the fitness goal fanatically, we make an idol out of it. I believe this should be apparent to Christians whether or not we regard the promotion of excessive exercise as arising from the New Age movement.

Vegetarianism is considered by some to be another potential area of concern. Before I offend some readers I should perhaps point out that vegetarianism is a major component of Hinduism and the Hare Krishna cult, to name just two movements. The Hindu faith forbids Hindus in India to eat cows because they are sacred. Ironically, it has been estimated that, were the cows eaten rather than fed, India's famine problem could be obliterated. Various animal rights groups have embraced the vegetarian theme and some of their literature is steeped in New Age influence, with liberal use of such terms as 'Mother Earth'.

For some, their upbringing or natural inclination may mean that a vegetarian lifestyle seems irresistible. Like exercise, there is always some truth in the philosophy. There is scientific evidence to support the view that people in western societies generally eat too much fat and protein and not enough fibre. It is part of biblical teaching that God gave mankind responsibility to care for the earth and its resources. On the whole we have made a poor job of it, and Christians should be concerned with environmental issues.

However, the Bible teaches that, after the changes in climate which followed the flood, God gave 'everything that lives and moves' as food for mankind.[16] If we refute

God's provision for us, on the grounds that by doing so we are being kinder to animals or adopting a healthier life-style, we need to be sure that we are not rejecting God's order in creation and making idols out of the animal kingdom or our own health.

Ironically, there is a high incidence of iron-deficiency anaemia in women of child-bearing age who eat a vege-tarian diet containing little available iron. Furthermore, it is interesting that the better established and more tradi-tional animal welfare societies avoid these issues. They rightly work towards goals that we should all support, such as humane breeding establishments, abattoirs and livestock transportation.

There are many more issues that could be discussed. They include the belief that cancer can be prevented by certain faddish diets (not borne out by epidemiological research), an obsession with stress and stress manage-ment, and preoccupation with various forms of medita-tion. In each case a valuable truth has been distorted. A balanced diet containing fruit, vitamins and minerals is beneficial to one's health, knowledge of relaxation tech-niques can be helpful, and in our rather hectic lifestyle it can be useful to reconsider the place of times of stillness. However, when the truth is distorted, pursuit of our own happiness becomes of paramount importance and these goals become what the Bible calls idols.

There can be a tendency for some Christians to blame the New Age for any and everything. I feel this is unhelp-ful. For one thing, as I said previously, the New Age is most definitely not new, although its proponents would like us to think it is because it always sounds much more attractive that way. Secondly, by blaming the New Age movement, Christians are absolved from the responsibility to think. Provided they can label something as 'New Age', they can reject it. What will they do when the New Age disappears (as it will) and the same heresies appear under a different name? Christians need to use their minds and not be too naive.

Dr George Smith, general practitioner and dermatologist, reports that Christians have suffered what one might label spiritual side-effects from involvement in yoga and TM.[17] He lists anxiety, depression, fear, lack of Christian assurance, interference with prayer life and Bible reading and demonic oppression amongst possible hazards, but does not cite specific examples.

It will probably never be possible to document with precision these more subtle hazards associated with alternative medicine. However, it should be of concern to Christians that alternative remedies with a psychic basis often involve the worship of other gods. As such they are forbidden by God.[18]

We can conclude that there will always be the need for Christians to explore whether there is a psychic basis to a particular alternative therapy. Only after investigating this should we carefully and prayerfully consider whether to embark on such therapy.

5

FACT OR FICTION?

Science is nothing but trained and organized common sense
T.H. Huxley *Collected Essays*

What is truth?

John 18:38

In the introduction we outlined why the issue of alternative medicine cannot be ignored. In chapter one we discovered that some treatments available on the NHS, such as psychotherapy, have not always been as thoroughly evaluated as one might expect. We could therefore not define alternative medicine as all practices which have not been subjected to rigorous evaluation, and had to use instead definitions of orthodox and alternative medicine based on the current medical school curriculum. In chapter two we looked briefly at the historical background to orthodox and alternative medicine. In chapter three we examined why alternative medicine has become so much more popular in recent years. In chapter four we looked at some of the treatments which make up alternative medicine and examined the potential problems associated with their unrestricted practice.

Evaluating Treatment

In order to advance the frontiers of medical knowledge, doctors and scientists can never be satisfied with the status quo. New treatments must continually be developed and evaluated. Objective evaluation of new treatments is always an extremely demanding challenge. The need for proper evaluation, possible ways of doing this, and some of the potential problems encountered, are outlined in this chapter.

I will begin by discussing the methods which doctors and medical scientists currently use to evaluate medical (and surgical) treatments of many varieties. So far such methods have been largely applied to orthodox medicine, the most striking recent exception being that of osteopathy.

Why Evaluate?

It is important that medical therapies offered to the public should be known to be effective, whether their cost is subsidised by the government or charged directly to the individual. Ineffective treatments waste the patient's time and money and may mean that the patient is denied another genuinely effective remedy. New treatments must also be shown to be safe, or at least safer than the existing ones.

Drug Development

Drug discovery arises in various ways. As discussed previously, a compound may be developed from herbal remedies, examples being morphine and digoxin. Sometimes good fortune, coupled with detailed observation and hard work, are responsible. An example is the discovery of penicillin by Alexander Fleming.

Alternatively, drugs may be developed rationally on the basis of existing knowledge and hypotheses about the cause of disease. Such a drug is L-dopa, used to treat Parkinson's disease. Prior to its development, it was known that there were reduced amounts of dopamine in the brains of patients with Parkinsonism. L-dopa is converted to dopamine following administration to the patient. The rationale for using it was therefore to restore levels of dopamine to normal.

Drug Testing

Once a potential drug is discovered it undergoes extensive pharmacological testing to determine its therapeutic properties and potential side-effects. When enough is known about its safety, it is given to healthy volunteers and its effects recorded. If it is found to be safe, short-term studies are then performed on patients, followed by large-scale ones possibly conducted over a longer period of time. Only after satisfying these stages is a new drug released onto the market.

Throughout the world, and especially in 'developed' countries, there exist drug regulatory authorities whose task is to ensure that drugs are of acceptable quality, efficacy and safety. In the UK this responsibility lies with the Health Ministers for England and Wales, Scotland and Northern Ireland. These ministers form the Licensing Authority which issues licences and certificates for new drugs. In this way, every effort is made to ensure that only safe and effective drugs reach the public.

The Medicines Division of the Department of Health was restructured in 1989. This established the Medicines Control Agency (MCA) as an agent of the licensing authority. The MCA has the power and responsibility to ensure that legal requirements concerning the manufacture, sale and promotion of drugs are met. The Committee on Safety of Medicines is the body to which all licence applications for new drugs have to be submitted and advises the MCA on whether a drug should be licensed for clinical trial and subsequent marketing.

Old treatments are continuously being challenged by

newer ones. For doctors, it is deciding whether these newer treatments are an improvement over established ones that often presents the greatest challenge.

Clinical Trials

Sometimes it is relatively easy to demonstrate the efficacy of a given treatment. The more predictable the outcome of the disease, and the more effective the treatment, the easier it is to prove. For example, the efficacy of penicillin in treating pneumococcal pneumonia is dramatic and easy to prove. However, striking results such as these are relatively uncommon in medicine and some kind of formal study is needed to evaluate therapies. By subjecting both orthodox medicine to more rigorous evaluation, and examining alternative medicine in this way, we will be better enabled to discover which treatments are of genuine value in fighting disease.

The placebo effect, as discussed previously, is the term given to describe the observation that one third of all people, given an inert compound to relieve a particular symptom, will report relief of that symptom. Owing to this phenomenon it is often not easy to determine whether a particular treatment is effective. Clinical trials help doctors to evaluate new therapies more objectively.

How do we define whether a particular treatment is effective? We may state that it should be shown to alleviate one or more symptoms, or to ameliorate or cure a disease. Which symptoms we define as important will be determined both by our understanding of the natural history of the disease and by the patient's expectations. Two examples given below illustrate this.

In treating a patient with terminal cancer and a life expectancy of only a few days we may choose to give a drug which successfully relieves pain, even though we know that it could under some circumstances shorten life. In this situation the patient's quality of life becomes of greater importance than its length in days or weeks.

However, when evaluating a new treatment for heart attack we will want to examine its effect on survival after one, six or twelve months. We will probably also want to investigate its effect on the functioning of the heart muscle and efficiency of blood flow in the coronary arteries at various times after the heart attack. Thus in order to assess the efficacy of a given treatment in this situation we need to know first what measurements will accurately predict long-term survival, as well as considering the patient's quality of life when it is prolonged.

In any one individual who receives a particular treatment the benefit of treatment should outweigh any likely hazard, or risk, associated with the treatment. Whenever doctors prescribe drugs or perform surgical procedures they have to make some assessment of the benefit:risk ratio to the individual patient.

As mentioned previously, subjective impressions of whether a particular treatment is effective are known to be potentially misleading. This is partly because both doctors and patients tend to be biased towards believing that the treatment is beneficial, and partly because of the placebo phenomenon.

A clinical trial involves the administration of one or more therapies to a group of individuals under medical supervision. There has to be some pre-existing evidence suggesting that the treatment may be beneficial, and the study should demonstrate both efficacy and side-effects the therapy may have. It can be applied to procedures (for example a surgical operation) as well as to the administration of a drug.

At its simplest, a clinical trial may compare the efficacy and safety of two drugs, A and B. Alternatively it may compare a drug A with a placebo. The placebo is usually an inert compound with no pharmacological activity. A brief outline of some of the issues which need to be considered by doctors performing clinical trials is given below.

Numbers of patients

The study is usually carried out in a substantial number of patients. This is because all individuals are unique, and will therefore respond slightly differently to the same treatment. It is thus always potentially possible to claim that a new treatment is valuable if it has only been given to one or two patients. The number of patients required depends partly upon the expected difference in efficacy between treatments. If treatment A improves outcome by 10%, a substantial number of patients will be needed to confirm that it confers an advantage over existing treatments. If, however, treatment A is thought to improve outcome by 50%, fewer patients will be required to demonstrate the beneficial effect.

Bias

An investigator who knows which treatment a patient is receiving may in some way, even unconsciously, influence the outcome because his or her judgement is biased. In order to try and eliminate such bias in a study, clinical trials are whenever possible performed in a 'double-blind' manner. This means that neither the doctor nor the patient knows which treatment the patient is receiving until after the study is finished. Furthermore, patients are usually randomly allocated to each treatment group, hence the term 'randomised' controlled trial.

Ethics

A number of ethical issues have to be addressed in clinical trials. Examples include using uncomfortable or potentially hazardous procedures which would not normally be needed in the course of investigation or treatment and the use of a placebo where there already exists a drug thought to be effective.

The question of what constitutes 'informed consent' is particularly difficult. Where patients are asked to undergo surgery, diagnostic procedures, or take part in medical research, they are required to give what is termed 'informed consent'. The idea is that the patient should be fully aware of the nature of the procedure, and of the risks involved. In practice, most risks are extremely rare, and there will only be one or two complications which commonly arise. If one were to list all the possible risks involved in having one's appendix removed, very many patients would probably have serious doubts about the advisability of proceeding! In reality, the risks are usually extremely small. It is therefore often difficult to know how far to go in trying to explain all the details, including very remote hazards, to patients.

Clinical trials in conditions where the patients may be elderly, suffering from mental illness or children, pose extra difficulties. Owing to these difficulties, all research centres and hospitals carrying out clinical trials have independent ethical committees to examine all clinical research proposals and advise whether they consider them to be ethical. Such committees include lay members of the public as well as healthcare professionals.

Given the above considerations, it is clear that clinical trials cannot be undertaken lightly and are often complex to plan and perform. In some cases several clinical trials, designed to answer the same question, produce conflicting results. This is because a large number of variables can affect the outcome of a clinical trial. These include the precise question the trial was designed to answer, the number and characteristics of the subjects studied, the dose and method of administration of the drug(s) given or the experience of the surgeon(s) involved in performing a surgical procedure, the length of treatment, the outcome measures chosen (for example death, survival at one year or the patient's perception of quality of life), the length of follow-up after cessation of treatment, and the methods used for statistical analysis. Clinical trials are almost invariably performed in a variety of countries with a number of different variables such as those mentioned above, and not infrequently yield apparently contradictory conclusions. Doctors are then left in a real dilemma as to which body of evidence they can trust.

Scientific Evaluation of Alternative Therapies

So far we have examined the ways in which doctors and clinical scientists attempt to evaluate the safety and efficacy of both new and existing treatments. I believe both the medical profession and alternative practitioners must attempt to evaluate alternative therapies using the same methods that are currently applied to orthodox therapies.

However, in applying the use of clinical trials to alternative therapies, difficulties arise. For instance, it is obviously impossible to conduct a double-blind trial comparing manipulative (osteopathic or chiropractic) therapy with non-manipulative therapy. Nevertheless, as a recent Lancet editorial highlighted,[1] trials do not necessarily have to be performed in the traditional double-blind fashion to yield valuable information.

An extract from this editorial reads, 'To carry scientific credibility, patients receiving a new treatment must be tested against a very similar control group who receive either the current standard treatment or no active treatment at all. Allocation to each group must be rigorously randomised. When the outcome is objective and completely independent of judgement by the subject or by the trialist' [for example, survival] 'blinding of either is not crucial.' When physical treatments are being assessed, the alternative treatment can be compared with a conventional treatment (such as physiotherapy) that can be applied with equal conviction, time and attention given to each individual.

Despite such limitations, I believe clinical trials will be an essential tool in evaluating new treatments. Trial results should be repeatable and independent of any 'magical' powers claimed by the practitioner. Such studies will lead the way forward in furthering our understanding about the way such treatments work and their effectiveness.

Alternative Therapies on Trial

In this section I will consider some examples of instances where controlled trials have already been performed to evaluate some alternative therapies.

A large randomised trial conducted by the Medical Research Council compared chiropractic and orthodox treatment of low back pain.[2] A recent review of clinical trials in homoeopathy[3] concluded that evidence of definitive benefit from homoeopathic remedies was at present still lacking because most of the trials were not sufficiently well designed. Double-blind studies could potentially be carried out to evaluate homoeopathic remedies, and the review recommends that a few well-designed trials involving large numbers of patients should be performed.

A number of studies have evaluated the use of acupuncture, both in the UK, Europe and China. There is some evidence that the release of the body's own pain-relieving chemicals (endorphins) is increased following acupuncture and may contribute to pain relief.[4] A number of studies have recorded objective physiological effects during acupuncture resulting in a diminished awareness of pain (termed an increased pain threshold). This therefore provides a scientific basis on which to conduct further research and clinical trials. A recent study which examined the use of electroacupuncture (where traditional acupuncture needles are connected to an electric current after insertion) in the treatment of fibromyalgia showed significant benefit.[5]

There have been few controlled trials evaluating the use of herbal remedies, despite the large number of reports of their toxicity. Data on other alternative therapies is equally sparse and further studies are required. An example of an encouraging response to current trends is provided by a recent study of the effect of oil of evening primrose on menopausal flushing.[6]

The symptoms experienced by many women at the onset of menopause are effectively treated by oestrogen supplements but some women cannot tolerate hormone replacement therapy or prefer not to take it. In these patients symptoms remain troublesome. The rationale for performing this study is stated by the authors as follows 'Although neither clinicians nor the pharmaceutical industry have ever promoted evening primrose oil for the purpose, there is a current view among the lay public that it is effective in the control of menopausal vasomotor symptoms', ie flushing.

They go on, 'Anecdotal cases have been reported supporting this in some menopausal women taking preparations of evening primrose oil. Consequently, large quantities of the oil in various formulations are being bought over the counter. In view of the possible theoretical benefits of the oil and the fact that it is being widely used by women in the general population its efficacy in suppressing adverse climacteric symptoms needs to be formally assessed.'

The authors proceeded to conduct a randomised, double blind, placebo controlled pilot study in thirty-five women. There was no significant benefit of evening primrose oil over placebo and the authors concluded that there is at present no evidence to support the use of evening primrose oil in treating menopausal hot flushes. Such studies are extremely valuable and should be applied to other popular remedies. However, the companies who promote these products may not fund such studies. The market for evening primrose oil was £17m in 1991 and £36m in 1993,[7] and a pot of sixty capsules in 1995 costs around £5.90.

A four year trial of the use of beta-carotene, vitamins C and E and placebo in the prevention of large bowel tumours showed no beneficial protective effect. Another report has been published showing no protective effect of vitamins on the development of lung cancer.[8]

Regulation of Alternative Therapies

Where an alternative therapy has been validated by such studies, regulation of alternative practitioners and their remedies is then necessary.

Regulation within each field of alternative therapy should include four elements.

1. Register   There should be a register of all members. It should be open to public scrutiny and entry to the register should be limited to competent practitioners.

2. Code of Conduct   There should be guidelines regarding the professional standards required, competence to practise, and ethical conduct.

3. Core Curriculum   There should be a formal training structure with a core curriculum.

4. Basic Medical Science Training   Training in the basic medical sciences should be compulsory. Alternative practitioners should be aware of the limits of their competence and be taught to diagnose conditions which are contra-indications to the treatment they offer.

For example, osteopaths should be able to recognise signs suggestive of a bone tumour and a massage thera-pist should be able to recognise signs suggestive of deep venous thrombosis. In both cases, the condition is not amenable to alternative therapy and may worsen, with hazardous consequences, if not treated by conventional medical and/or surgical methods. There should be clear protocols for communicating with medical practitioners and therapists should be prevented from revoking instruc-tions or prescriptions given by a doctor. A case was reported where a homoeopath instructed his client to halve the dose of blood pressure medication prescribed for him by his general practitioner.[9] Finally, research and professional development should be encouraged.

One example of how regulation of alternative therapies might be conducted in the future is given below. In March 1994, following a European Union homoeopathic direc-tive incorporated into UK law the preceding month, the MCA set up a Homoeopathic Registration Scheme.

Regulations now exist to harmonise the manufacture, control and supply of homoeopathic products throughout the European Union (EU). In order to be eligible for registration, manufacturers will have to produce evidence of the pharmaceutical quality of their product. Homoeo-pathic remedies should satisfy a number of criteria.

They should be prepared from recognised homoeopathic stocks in accordance with a homoeopathic manufacturing procedure described by a pharmacopoeia used within the EU. They should be for oral or external use only (that is they should not be intended for injection). There should be no specific therapeutic indication included in the product labelling or information sheet.

Each product must carry the scientific name of the stock from which it is prepared, and not a proprietary (trade) name. It should be sufficiently dilute to guarantee safety, containing no more than one part per 10,000 of the original tincture. Where the active ingredient is usually only available on prescription it should contain no more than one part per 100 of the lowest dose used in conventional medicines.

Other regulations have been introduced. Manufacturers of homoeopathic medicines, wholesale dealers and importers from non-EU countries will have to apply for licences.

Homoeopathic medicines which have been issued with a registration certificate may carry an HR registration number on the label. Only information specified in labelling requirements will be allowed in advertising the product. Advertising suggesting that health could be enhanced will be prohibited, and a warning will be given that the user should consult a doctor if symptoms persist during use of the product.

Two very important exemptions exist. Firstly, it is notable that evidence of efficacy is still not required under this registration scheme. Thus compounds are still being actively marketed when there is no firm evidence that they are beneficial.

Secondly, manufacturers of products covered by old product licences can continue to market their products. However, homoeopathic remedies not authorised by any form of registration will only be sold or supplied on a 'named patient basis' and will thus not be for sale to the general public.

Similar steps are being taken in the USA. New labelling methods introduced by the Food and Drug Administration in 1994 will make it more difficult for the manufacturers of vitamins and other dietary supplements to make health claims on behalf of their products. Declarations printed on labels now have to be supported by 'significant agreement among qualified experts'.[10]

In Britain, registration will help to ensure that these

remedies will not cause harm. However, registration alone is obviously not sufficient to guarantee that a given remedy is beneficial and there remains an urgent need for clinical trials to establish or disprove the efficacy of such treatments.

For details of other procedures that could be followed to regulate alternative therapies, the reader is referred to the recent recommendations set out by the BMA.[11]

In this chapter I have illustrated ways in which conventional methods could be applied more widely to evaluate and regulate certain alternative therapies. In chapter six I will examine some practical ways in which individual Christians might evaluate such therapies. I will also consider what specific responses Christian doctors might make to the challenges posed by alternative medicine.

6

A CHRISTIAN RESPONSE

Beware that you do not lose the substance by grasping at the shadow.

> Aesop's Fables: 'The Dog and The Shadow'

Test everything. Hold on to the good.

> 1 Thessalonians 5:21

Medicine and the Bible

Before discussing a possible Christian response to alternative therapies I want to consider briefly what the Bible has to say about medicine. Despite many references in the Bible to sin, sickness, health and healing, there are few direct references to medical practice.

Much of the Old Testament describes the history of the Jewish nation. During Joseph's life his family, seventy people in all, settled in Egypt. Later, under a new ruler (Pharaoh), their descendants, the Israelites, were forced into slavery. Alarmed by the continued expansion of these foreigners in his country, the Pharaoh ordered that the midwives should kill all baby boys born into Jewish families. Two midwives who disobeyed his command are commended and blessed by God.[1] This clearly endorses the view that all life is precious in God's eyes and that infanticide is wrong. It also makes it clear that God's people relied on the midwives and medical practitioners of their day just as their neighbours did, and that God sanctioned this.

There is a brief reference to the part our mental state can play in our physical health in the book of Proverbs,[2] where it states that a 'cheerful heart is good medicine'. No-one, I am sure, would disagree with this commonsense statement.

The Apocrypha is a collection of writings considered to contain teaching which is edifying for the church but lacks the divine authority of the rest of Scripture. Ecclesiasticus is a collection of writings giving practical advice for life. In this book, medical skill is seen as God's gift[3]: 'Honour the physician with the honour due to him, according to your need of him, for the Lord created him; for healing comes from the Most High...The Lord created medicines from the earth, and a sensible man will not despise them...he gave skill to men that he might be glorified in his marvellous works. By them he heals and takes away pain...'

The writer of the third gospel, Luke, was a doctor by profession.[4] Not surprisingly, he sometimes includes medical details omitted in the other gospels. In his account he records Jesus healing a woman of a haemorrhage.[5] He says with sober realism, 'And a woman was there who had been subject to bleeding for twelve years, but no-one could heal her.' Doctors failed in those days just as they do now, but Jesus was able to heal her.

What can we learn from these references? Firstly, that only God has the power to give or withhold healing. All healing should therefore be regarded as being divine in origin. Secondly, in His compassion, God has entrusted some medical knowledge and skills as a gift to mankind. Consequently He expects His people to consult doctors.

Thirdly, it is recognised that there will probably be numerous conditions which doctors are unable to cure.

In practice, I believe these considerations mean several things. Christians should be careful not to reject medicine or its practitioners just because they do not always share their beliefs. Faith in God is not required to exercise these skills, and many brilliant and compassionate doctors have been, are and always will be, atheists or agnostics.

Christians can help those who have fallen into the trap of thinking that conventional medicine will always be successful. Doctors fail, treatments fail, and patients remain ill or die. As we have seen, many today expect instant and complete cures, and so are disappointed. Christians have the opportunity to point them to an all-powerful, all-loving God, but they must remember that God's omnipotence and benevolence do not guarantee us physical or psychological health in this life. When He does not heal, His love and presence remain with us to support us.

A Christian Response To Alternative Medicine

There is evidently a need for objectivity about orthodox medicine. What about alternative medicine? There are four general questions we can ask about any new therapy being offered and I have outlined them below.

Facts

Do the claims for this therapy fit the facts? Some answers to this question are not as difficult for a layperson to find as one might think.

In some cases publicity is obviously misleading. It does not require medical qualifications to spot this type of publicity once made aware of it. While not necessarily associated with occult practices, such publicity is blatantly untruthful. Examples are claims that one form of treatment will cure a vast number of diseases. Such publicity comes in leaflets distributed in a variety of ways.

One such pamphlet I received recently reads as follows: 'This is a guide to a much wider range of ailments which can be treated ...**Pains of all kinds:** arthritis, sciatica, tennis elbow, back pain, tendenitis [misspelt], headache, trigeminal neuralgia, lumbago. **Disorders:** Infections – bronchitis, cold, flu, Ear nose and throat – hay fever, sinusitis, tinitus [misspelt], Alimentary – duodenal ulcer, indigestion, gastric ulcers, obesity, haemorrhoids, Circulatory – anaemia, palpitations, high/low blood pressure, Pulmonary – bronchiectasis, Dermatological – acne, psoriasis, eczema, herpes, Genito-Urinary & Reproductive – dysmenorrhoea, menopausal symptoms, impotence, menstrual disorder, cystitis, Endoctrinal [misspelt] – hormonal problem, adrenal insufficiency, Mental-Emotional – anxiety, insomnia, depression, periperhal neuritis, stress, Other Problems – smoking, weight, alcoholism'.

Not only is this list ridiculously extensive, it is also a quite random selection of disorders, some of which overlap. A slightly less obviously deceptive list, more worrying because all the more believable, was provided by a bogus doctor jailed in June 1993 for issuing a misleading advertisement.[6] She styled herself as a professor despite having no medical qualifications and recruited volunteers for her 'new product', called CH6 or Cancelle.

Analysis by chemists showed that it contained toxic elements and had no medicinal properties. In her booklet, emotively titled 'Cancer and AIDS: Is There Any Hope Left For Us?', she claimed that CH6 could cure cancer, 'eliminate the HIV virus 100%' and treat Parkinson's disease, myalgic encephalitis, hepatitis, cystic fibrosis, arthritis, sickle cell anaemia, haemophilia, herpes, meningitis, multiple sclerosis and asthma.

What is particularly worrying about this type of advertising is that nearly all these disorders are serious conditions often only partly amenable to conventional treatment. Those who have had any contact with sufferers of any one of these diseases will know how desperate such patients are for any new treatment which will improve their condition. The first example was merely laughable; this one is more serious because it uses emotionally sensitive language. In reality, one drug is never the solution for all diseases, although it may indeed have several applications.

Scientific Basis

It is important to establish whether there is any scientific basis for the therapy on offer. The practitioner offering treatment should be able and willing to provide this kind of information. If they are not, it should alert us to the possibility that either they themselves are not competent or else that the treatment has no scientific basis. If it has no scientific basis, we must bear in mind that it may not be harmless. As I have illustrated previously, even apparently innocuous substances may have harmful physical side-effects. Alternatively it may be based on a psychic form of healing. If we are in doubt regarding the validity of scientific claims, we should be able to consult our general practitioner about the treatment.

The Therapist's World-view

Behind some (but not all) alternative therapies on offer today there lies a hidden, spiritual agenda. How do we recognise this and how should we respond?

Christians are to avoid treatments which are associated with occult practices. By occult practices I mean practices characterised by mystical or supernatural phenomena. As mentioned previously, God makes it very clear in the Old Testament that His people are to have no dealings whatsoever with spiritualists or mediums of any kind.[7] This is because the Bible recognises the existence of evil and does not dismiss it lightly. However, sometimes one therapy can be offered by two different practitioners with wholly opposing views and beliefs. Consider the case of acupuncture, which illustrates this very clearly.

Several articles have been written by evangelical Christians denouncing acupuncture as a work of the devil to be avoided at all costs. A number of equally evangelical Christians have studied acupuncture in some depth and have come to opposite conclusions.

Why is there such a difference of opinion? The former Christians have denounced acupuncture on the basis that it is connected with the occult. However, the word occult can also be used to describe phenomena beyond ordinary human understanding, or not at present explicable in western scientific terms. This is not the meaning given in the Bible[8] where it is involved with evil spirits and divination which are clearly condemned.

The practice and theory of acupuncture date back to at least 540 BC in China. The theory put forward to explain the basis of acupuncture was as follows. As mentioned in chapter two, life was thought to be dependent on a combination in specific proportions of yang (energy from the sun) and yin (energy from the earth). Sickness was attributed to an imbalance of these two energies.

Health was thought to be maintained by movement of the vital breath in channels between the various vital organs. These channels were thought to run in lines up and down the body, named after the organ they served and often depicted on models as lines or meridians. The models served merely as anatomy models to demonstrate the various lines and anatomy points. It was thought that it was possible to influence the movement of this vital force and restore the normal flow by stimulating these channels at certain points along their course using needles.

A traditional acupuncturist will work on this basis and may well also prescribe herbal medicine and give advice about diet. A modern acupuncturist, often a western doctor, will take a straightforward history, formulate a diagnosis in traditional western medical terms, may not believe in the existence of meridians and may find his own acupuncture points. Fine disposable injection needles are as effective as traditional acupuncture needles.

The traditional Chinese view of health and disease differs from our own. However, there is no association between acupuncture in traditional Chinese medicine and seeking help from outside spiritual forces, consulting astrological charts or signs or any type of fortune-telling.

The controversy has probably arisen because in some cases Christians have failed to realise that a people's basic philosophy of life will determine that people's interpretation in all areas of life, whether their experiences be good, bad or neutral in themselves. Any phenomena in any society, whether they be earthquakes, diseases, famines or droughts, are open to spiritual explanation. The phenomenon of acupuncture was discovered in a non-Christian culture and interpreted in a non-Christian framework.

We can reject the traditional interpretation of acupuncture because we now have some knowledge of how it may work in physiological terms, but this does not mean that we have to reject acupuncture itself.

In reality, the concept of health being a balance of opposing forces is not unusual or particularly non-Christian. As we saw earlier, the Greeks proposed that illness resulted from an imbalance of the four basic humours, and this theory was held to be valid until the mid-19th century. Similar concepts operate in western medicine today. Autonomic nervous function is considered to be maintained by a balance between opposing sympathetic and parasympathetic systems. Muscle groups are categorised into opposing groups, hormones are described as having opposite and thus balancing actions, and there is considered to be a critical acid-base balance in the body.

What is obviously contrary to Christian belief is the Chinese philosophy that the source of all life is the Tao ('the way'), that the whole cosmos is interrelated and that man remains healthy by attuning himself to the balance of the cosmos. We can and should reject this philosophy, but we should bear in mind that all events, including the year's seasons, work and marriage were seen within this philosophy. Just as we do not reject the concepts of seasons, work and marriage because we reject this ancient non-Christian philosophy, we do not on this basis have to reject acupuncture.

Consider two modern-day acupuncturists. The first may be a consultant anaesthetist in a busy district general hospital, trying to give a patient with severe, unremitting pain some short-term relief. The second may be a spiritualist, or 'healer' whose treatment is only part of a programme involving the frankly occult. Christians need to be discerning enough to distinguish between these two types of treatment on offer. The above example is obviously clear-cut; others will in real life be less so. If in doubt, a few simple questions asked of the practitioner should quickly reveal his or her viewpoint.

There is medical evidence that acupuncture is beneficial under certain circumstances. In these circumstances I think it should be received as part of God's gifts. Where there is a spiritual association it should be rejected.

Motives:

The Therapist
Christians believe in the existence of evil and consequently in the existence of sin. Trying to live with the consequences of our own, and others' sin, in this world, is a challenge facing Christians and non-Christians alike. No one would pretend that it is ever possible to have absolutely pure motives for one's actions. Indeed, even impure motives can be harnessed for good. Desire for money or

prestige can drive someone to the heights of their chosen career and service to others. Nevertheless, I think that there are some principles that can be set out when examining motives behind alternative therapies.

An overwhelming desire for money, prestige or power may lie behind the more dubious practices now offered. There is obviously nothing wrong in a practitioner charging a reasonable fee for his or her services, but if the fee seems extortionate, we should perhaps consider again what is really the motive behind this so-called treatment.

It has been suggested that the success of some alternative therapists results from money changing hands. As one writer puts it, 'When we invest hard earned cash in a course of treatment, and with it a little bit of ego, we are that much more likely to view the results in a positive light to justify the expense'.[9] He goes on to suggest that the popularity of alternative medicine would decline if it were made available free on the NHS. It is generally true that when genuinely effective and safe treatments are being offered by alternative practitioners, money will not be their prime concern, but rather the well-being of patients.

In exactly the same way, the greater the desire for publicity, fame or power, the more likely it is that the treatment on offer is doubtful in its safety or efficacy. The General Medical Council (GMC), which in this country regulates doctors' professional conduct, restricts the rights of doctors to advertise.

An example of a case where desire for fame and money was apparently of greater importance than safety or efficacy of the treatment was reviewed recently.[10] This doctor practised medicine for only two years after qualifying. Nine years later he opened an allergy clinic. In 1993 he was found guilty by the GMC of touting for patients using a publicity agent, and of injecting a patient with a substance he knew would harm him.

A letter to his publicity agent reads: 'Herewith the letter

from Mrs Massey. I think you will agree it's got the beginnings of a nice story. To re-emphasise, I would like this one played a little bit special if you can. Try to get it as a 'Dr [X] does it again', not just a patient story. The effect from the *Sunday Express* article is just beginning to wane slightly and a boost now would be absolutely terrific and see us right through to Christmas.' It only takes commonsense to see that the motive behind this man's practice was not just the well-being of patients. Furthermore, the techniques of 'clinical ecology' which he used have not been scientifically validated.

Motives:

The Patient

We have seen that conventional medicine often fails to bring a cure or even relief for a large number of patients suffering from a variety of diseases. It is right that research should continue to pursue new avenues of treatment.

However, it is the view of some Christians in the more extreme charismatic sections of the church that, because sickness results from sin in the world, and because God is all-powerful and all-loving, it is never God's will for us to be ill. Failure to be healed is therefore attributed to sin or unbelief on the part of the patient.

I have seen the appalling devastation this teaching can bring to patients already suffering from dreadful diseases. I have heard the anguish of teenagers and university students when, facing premature death from the inherited disease cystic fibrosis, they are exposed to this cruel lie. David Watson recounts his distress associated with facing a similar situation when dying of bowel cancer.[11] He had at least the benefit of being older, wiser, and nearer the natural end of his life.

Christian leaders must exercise responsibility, sensitivity and caution in these areas. Otherwise they may be guilty of destroying the faith of children and other vulnerable, hurting people.

What does the Bible say about this issue of healing? We have seen that the Bible is clear that God can always heal, in whatever way He chooses. However, there is no guarantee that He always will in this life. Jesus's followers were not always able to heal the sick.[12] Paul had to leave his friend Trophimus unwell at Miletus[13] and was apparently unable to heal his colleague Epaphroditus, even though the latter nearly died of his illness.[14] Paul advised Timothy to use a little wine as a medicine when suffering from 'frequent illnesses'.[15] Paul himself suffered from illness.[16] He also refers to a 'thorn in my flesh' which God did not remove.[17]

Michael Green makes the point that it should not surprise us if God does not always heal us physically. He says, 'How people would rush to Christianity (and for all the wrong motives) if it carried with it automatic exemption from sickness! What a nonsense it would make of Christian virtues like longsuffering, patience and endurance. . . What a wrong impression it would give of salvation if physical wholeness were perfectly realised on earth whilst spiritual wholeness were partly reserved for heaven! What a very curious thing it would be if God were to decree death for all his children whilst not allowing illness for any of them!'[18]

We do not know why God allows suffering in this world. No-one should pretend to have all the answers. What Christians hold onto is that Jesus Christ, by allowing Himself to be crucified, took part in our physical and spiritual anguish. We are never alone in our suffering. Perhaps the Church needs to re-develop a theory of suffering, without denying the wonderful deeds that God can and does perform in the 20th century.

As Christians we therefore need to examine our own motives when seeking alternative therapies. Is our highest priority to honour God? Or have we fallen into that familiar trap of believing lies about God? We should always pray as we seek conventional treatment. The church also has a role to play.[19] If God does not heal us, and our suffering becomes unbearable, we may need to remember that Jesus knows the reality of excruciating physical pain.

A Christian Doctor's Response To Alternative Medicine

There are a number of areas where Christian doctors could play an active role in responding positively to the challenge presented by alternative therapies. These largely have to do with the reasons for the rise in its popularity, which we discussed in chapter three. I have outlined some suggestions below.

Greater Hope?

We need to be responsible in giving realistic expectations to our patients. This may be as a general practitioner, hospital clinician or in public broadcasting. Our enthusiasm for a particular new treatment must always be tempered with realism.

Greater Disappointment?

We must be honest about the prognosis in chronic disease. Obviously this does not mean we always have to tell the patient unwelcome news he or she does not want to hear, but we should encourage our patients to ask questions. We can all learn from the communication skills developed within the hospice movement, and we should never think that we have 'arrived' in this difficult area.

We should be honest about possible side-effects. It may not be appropriate to detail all the fine print, but frequent or serious complications should be discussed. Again, encouraging the patient to ask questions should enable any overriding concerns he or she may have to be aired.

As a profession, we need to look again at the support we give, or fail to give, to our patients. We need imaginative ways of saving time and delegating clerical and technical tasks. We may need to recruit non-medical staff to broaden the emotional support available for patients.

We should examine constructively ways in which the working patterns of junior doctors can be made compatible with quality of life. It has been said that junior doctors lack compassion because they work in a system which affords them no compassion. This is not surprising when many of their tasks are performed at times when they could not safely drive a car or fly a plane.

If doctors are to continue to provide a professional service to patients, consultants and general practitioners will need to retain some authority within the NHS. They will have to insist on having adequate numbers of qualified staff to perform the various tasks required. This will require prayer, imagination and wisdom.

Finally, we must ensure that the interests of future patients will be served by preserving high quality medical research. This may include delivering enthusiastic tuition to students, attracting dedicated graduates and publicising the need for adequate funding.

Society

We need to be sensitive to the special needs of ethnic minorities. We may need to employ more interpreters or set up special clinics where their interests are better met. We need to consider whether we are contributing to racial prejudice and possibly misogyny within the medical profession. Ethnic minorities and women need better representation in the higher échelons of medicine.

Inequalities in health care provision and accessibility should be recognised and dealt with in so far as we are able. For some of us this will mean dealing with personal prejudices, for others it may mean political involvement.

We need to reform paternalistic attitudes towards patients and defensiveness in the face of effective alternative therapies. The contempt in which the orthodox medical profession has held osteopaths for many years is an obvious example.

Christian doctors should support, and not despise, patients who want to know more about alternative therapies. They should however be ready to point out spiritual dangers as well as physical ones.

Finally, I believe that there is a growing section of the medical profession which is only too aware of the faults of previous generations of doctors and is trying to make amends by welcoming with open arms all alternative remedies. This has its own dangers. If Christian doctors will repent of past mistakes and then seek wisdom from God, He will surely help us to be discerning.

What About Prayer?

I have already alluded to the physical and psychological healing that God can bring to individuals in response to prayer in the context of the Christian church. Such healing may obviously occur independently of medical treatment, but it tends to be sporadic. It may be confirmed by medical experts. Christians are urged to pray, and as doctors we should support this teaching.

Yet the power of prayer cannot be reproduced or compared with conventional drugs in large clinical trials. I believe this will remain one of the paradoxes facing Christian doctors until the end of time. I do not believe there are any easy answers because, in the end, none of us can dictate to God. Jesus the Great Physician is also 'the Lion of the tribe of Judah'.[20]

Conclusion

It is unrealistic to expect that Christians will ever agree on all aspects of alternative medicine. Within the church they disagree openly on aspects such as the ordination of women and the role of the church in politics. My own views, outlined in this chapter, will doubtless not be accepted by all. It is part of the glory of God's creation that He made us all very different and that we do not respond to Him like robots. Having accepted the authority of the Bible, and the absolute truths it contains, we have to decide for ourselves what is right. Let us in humility consult the Bible, pray, think, and act, preferably with others. When we feel daunted we should recall God's promise that 'Never will I leave you; never will I forsake you'[21].

Part III

7

THE ESSENTIAL A TO Z GUIDE

In such a night Medea gathered the enchanted herbs
That did renew old Aeson.
                              Shakespeare *The Merchant of Venice*

I love fruit, when it is expensive.
                    Sir Arthur Pinero *Second Mrs Tanqueray, I.*

A

Acupuncture   This is traditionally a branch of Chinese medicine. Needles are inserted into the body just below the skin at various pre-defined points.

Alexander Technique   This technique is named after F. Matthias Alexander. Teaching is given to correct posture and faulty movement patterns, usually to relieve back or neck pain or headaches.

Aromatherapy   Massage is given with plant oils. Some of the oils can also be taken internally.

B

Bach Flower Remedies   Infusions are made from wild plants and trees and subsequently diluted. The infusions are then taken internally.

Biomagnetics   Magnets are applied to acupuncture meridians in the belief that they can induce spinal and pelvic alignment.

C

Chiropractic   Manipulation, massage and other joint-adjusting procedures are used to treat musculo-skeletal complaints. Emphasis is placed on the use of spinal X-rays to diagnose mechanical problems. It differs from osteopathy in making more extensive use of soft-tissue massage, exercises, corsets, splints and supports.

Crystal Healing This is a treatment based on the idea that certain crystals and gems have healing 'energies', which may be imparted by touch or meditation. Elixirs may also be given internally.

D

Dance Therapy This term covers a range of treatments, all of which involve the use of dance and music for healing.

E

Encounter Therapy This is a psychological treatment which emphasises physical expression as a route to 'self-actualisation' and inner growth.

F

Faith Healing This is an umbrella term. It includes all treatments which involve conviction on the part of the practitioner or 'healer' and very often the laying on of hands, in the belief that a healing energy or force can thereby be transmitted to the patient.

G

Ginseng This is the name given to either of two plants from China or North America, whose forked aromatic roots are thought to possess tonic and energy-giving properties. They are used medicinally.

H

Herbalism Plant or herb-based remedies are taken internally or applied as creams.

Homoeopathy This was formulated by Samuel Hahnemann (1755–1843) and based on simple remedies (exercise, nourishing diet and pure air) and two fundamental principles: *1. The Law of Similars* Diseases are cured by drugs which produce in healthy persons the symptoms found in those who are ill. *2. The Law of Infinitesimals* The smaller the dose, the more efficacious the medicine. A method of mixing, dilution and shaking was termed 'succussion' and the resulting preparation a 'potency'. The process of dilution and succussion is claimed by some to release a therapeutic 'immaterial and vital' force.

I

Iridology This is a method of diagnosis based on studying the markings on the irises of the eyes and observing changes in them.

K

Kinesiology Muscles are tested to gain information about the body. Light touch or firm pressure on 'reflex points' of the body are used together with diet to restore what is thought to be correct balance.

L

Lomi-Lomi A form of massage,

involving rubbing and kneading of areas of the body.

M

Mesotherapy Minute quantities of medication such as vitamins, muscle relaxants or calcium-regulating hormones are mixed with a local anaesthetic and injected into pre-defined points in the skin. It is thought that the subcutaneous layer acts a reservoir, slowly releasing the medication towards the target tissue over a period of several days.

N

Naturopathy The body's own natural healing is stimulated by a variety of treatments including herbal remedies and manipulation.

O

Orgonomy A form of therapy where healing energy is thought to be released from uninhibited sexual activity.

P

Polarity Therapy It is thought that there are five major centres in the body and that energy flows between these centres. Health is attributed to the free flow of energy between perfectly balanced centres.

Q

Quieting Reflex A method of self-hypnosis used in American schools to treat stress in children.

Children are told that stress occurs 'when parents get into the picture' and are told to go for advice instead to the 'wise men' who live inside their bodies. They are then taught to breathe slowly through imaginary holes in their feet.

R

Radionics This method uses instrumentation to provide specific corrective energies to the patient through contact, medication or broadcasting at a distance. It includes the practices of biomagnetics and signalysis therapy.

Reflexology Compression and massage are used at various 'reflex' points in the hands and feet.

S

Shiatsu A Japanese form of massage which uses finger pressure on hundreds of surface points of the body.

T

Transcendental Meditation A technique based on Hindu traditions. It is designed to relax and refresh the mind through the silent repetition of a 'mantra'. A mantra is a sacred word or syllable used as an object of concentration.

U

Unani An ancient system of

medicine and healing practised in Africa.

patients in NHS hospitals. It consists largely of mediums.

V

Visualisation Therapy A form of autosuggestion therapy involving the imagination. For example, a patient with cancer might be encouraged to relax, focus on breathing and to visualise or imagine the cancer under attack until it eventually disappears.

W

Witchcraft Not extinct. The Witchcraft Act was repealed in Britain in 1952. More recently the 'World Federation of Healers' was given approval to treat

Y

Yoga A Hindu system of philosophy which aims at the mystical union of the self with the Supreme Being in a state of complete awareness and tranquillity through a routine of physical and mental exercises.

Z

Zone Therapy Manipulation in certain zones of surface anatomy is said to have a healing effect on a distant organ with no known neurological pathway.

A Model for Assessment of Alternative Therapies

In chapter six I suggested some ways in which we could seek to evaluate new therapies being offered. I will now consider three different therapies, listed in the above A–Z, and illustrate how one might attempt to apply some specific questions to them. The aim of this exercise is to help the reader to develop his or her own ideas about how to assess alternative treatments. I have chosen these three because they are well known. The first two are particularly controversial, while the third illustrates how therapies based on non-Christian spiritual principles can be effective.

Two words of caution are needed here. Firstly, assumptions made in this book about the current state of scientific evidence for any one therapy will soon be outdated. Thus, what is thought to be fact today may not be fact tomorrow. Obviously this limitation does not apply to unchanging truths, such as the nature of God or evil, but it does mean that this model does not represent a set of unchanging rules.

Secondly, as I concluded in chapter six, God gives to us as individuals free choice. There are undoubtedly principles which God does not intend us to violate. I discussed some of these briefly in the introduction. We are not to murder or to steal. There is absolute truth. However, every individual is unique, with different personal circumstances and upbringing. There are also some questions to which we will never know the full answers in this life. On such controversial matters Paul wrote, '"Everything is permissible" – but not everything is beneficial. "Everything is permissible" – but not everything is constructive...So whether you eat or drink or whatever you do, do it all for the glory of God'.[1]

Acupuncture

1) *Do the Claims for this Therapy fit the Facts?*

The Council for Acupuncture offers acupuncture for a wide range of conditions including asthma and bronchitis, gastro-intestinal disorders, disease of the eye and mouth and neurological and musculoskeletal disorders. General practitioners commonly refer patients with chronic pain to pain clinics for acupuncture, but do not generally refer patients for acupuncture to treat other conditions.

Research into the effectiveness of acupuncture is carried out by this organisation, and the work has been published in a number of medical journals.

There is evidence that acupuncture can provide effective pain relief in certain conditions associated with chronic pain, particularly of musculoskeletal origin. At present there is less evidence that acupuncture is effective in other conditions. In asthma there appears to be some discernible benefit, but it is usually short-lived and less striking than the improvement seen with conventional treatment (see review).[2]

In the early 1970s a number of enthusiastic reports were published about the effectiveness of acupuncture in relieving addiction to heroin, alcohol and cigarette smoking. In 1991 an analysis of twenty-two controlled clinical studies concluded that the study designs were generally poor and the evidence did not support the view that acupuncture is effective in helping patients to stop cigarette smoking. For heroin and alcohol addiction the research was felt to be 'both scarce and of low quality'.[3]

It seems that for the other conditions listed, the jury is still out and further research is needed.

2) *Is There A Rational Scientific Basis For The Therapy?*

Objective physiological effects of acupuncture have been recorded when the needles are either manipulated after insertion or connected to an electric current (electroacupuncture). There is some evidence that acupuncture can be beneficial in pain relief. Electroacupuncture raises the pain threshold (ie. reduces the individual's sensitivity to pain) in dental pain, experimental pain due to heat and painful nerve stimulation.

How is it thought to work? Certain tender areas (trigger points) are found in association with some musculoskeletal or inflammatory conditions. If these areas are needled, the pain is temporarily relieved. There is a high degree of correlation between these points and the Chinese acupuncture points. The Gate theory, proposed by Melzack and Wall in 1965, suggested that stimulation of certain neural pathways blocked the input of painful stimuli. It is also known that electroacupuncture causes the release of the body's own morphine-like substances, which act as natural pain-killers.

In China, acupuncture is used to treat infectious disease, such as malaria and typhoid fever. It has been suggested that the toxicity of certain infectious diseases is in part mediated by the nervous system.[4] There might therefore be a quite rational explanation for a beneficial effect in these circumstances.

3) Is the Methodology or the Principle the Effective Element?

The question is, if it works, why? It would seem from the available evidence that, at least in terms of bringing pain relief, acupuncture works through as yet incompletely understood physiological principles.

4) What is the Therapist's World-view?

Following the discussion of acupuncture in chapter six, I concluded that we can reject the concepts of yang and yin without rejecting acupuncture.

5) Does the Therapy Involve the Occult?

As mentioned in chapter seven, there is no evidence that acupuncture is linked with seeking outside spiritual forces.

In conclusion, acupuncture may be effective in relieving pain, and there seems to be no physical or spiritual reason why it should not be used in this situation. Its benefit in other conditions is not well-established.

Homoeopathy

1) Do the Claims for this Therapy fit the Facts?

The Faculty of Homoeopathy, whose premises are based at the Royal London Homoeopathic Hospital, offers treatment for all conditions. Some research is carried out and published in medical journals such as the BMJ and the Lancet. Nevertheless, there are hardly any well-conducted clinical trials. Homoeopathic practitioners have sometimes been reluctant to pursue clinical trials on the grounds that their remedies are individual for each patient and therefore cannot be assessed in this way.

A trial published recently in the Lancet[5] suggested that a homoeopathic remedy might be of some benefit (albeit limited) in treating allergic asthma. The study was carefully conducted by doctors working at the Glasgow Royal Infirmary. The authors' results reproduced the findings of two previous studies and they conclude that there was 'evidence that homoeopathy does more than placebo'. They consider that the principles said to underly homoeopathy are irreconcilable with those of modern pharmacology, but speculate that electromagnetic or nuclear magnetic resonance changes may occur at high dilution and in some way underlie a biological activity.

2) Is There a Rational Scientific Basis for the Therapy?

At present, the answer has to be no. The above suggestions are purely speculative and remain to be refuted or confirmed.

3) Is the Methodology or the Principle the Effective Element?

As discussed above, there is at present scant evidence that homoeopathy is effective. Proponents have claimed that the process of dilution and shaking release a therapeutic force. Thus, if homoeopathy were in future shown to be effective, it might well be the methodology which was important.

4) What is the Therapist's World-view?

Hahnemann was a freemason and hypnotist but also an educated and compassionate practitioner in his day. Today, individual therapists have differing world-views.

5) *Does The Therapy Involve The Occult?*

Christians in the UK are divided about this issue. The answer to the question is not immediately obvious and depends on where the 'immaterial and vital' force is thought to originate from. This will depend to some extent on the therapist and their world-view. There is evidence from continental Europe of a link between homoeopathy and the occult. where it has been alleged that homoeopathic practitioners carry out research during séances and use occult practices such as the pendulum[6], but this is probably less common in Britain. Christian homoeopaths would of course not be involved in any such practices.

I would conclude that there is presently insufficient scientific evidence for homoeopathy for it to be a tenable therapy for the individual. Whether it will eventually gain scientific credibility remains to be seen. Given the isolated reports of an association with occult practices I would encourage the reader to be cautious and prayerful, and to make exhaustive enquiries if considering treatment.

Transcendental Meditation

1) *Do the Claims for this Therapy Fit the Facts?*

There is scientific evidence that transcendental meditation (TM) can produce benefits such as lowered blood pressure or reduced anxiety.

2) *Is there a Rational Scientific Basis for the Therapy?*

Deep breathing and meditation will reliably produce a state of relaxation, just as taking deep breaths before an examination may help to keep the candidate calm. The physiological changes are easily recorded.

3) Is the Methodology or the Principle the Effective Element?

In this instance it is not the principle of meditation (a specifically spiritual activity) which is effective, but the methodology of the technique. Any equally relaxing activity would produce the same physiological benefits.

4) What is the Therapist's World-view?

The therapist's world-view is based on Eastern philosophy and specifically Hindu concepts.

5) Does the Therapy Involve the Occult?

There is no overt occult association.

In conclusion, I believe that the association with the Hindu religion precludes Christians from taking part in this kind of meditation. Other, Christian forms of prayer and meditation may be helpful, or other ways of relieving stress in one's lifestyle may need to be explored.

REFERENCES

All Bible quotations are taken from the New International Version (1978, New York International Bible Society).

Introduction

1. Gumbel, N. Questions of Life. Kingsway: UK, 1993.
2. McDowell, J. Evidence That Demands A Verdict. Campus Crusade for Christ Inc.: USA, 1972.
3. Exodus 20:13.
4. Consumers Association. 'Magic or Medicine'. Which? (Oct 1986):pp 443–447.
5. Fisher, P. and Ward, A. BMJ (1994): 309:107–111.
6. Karcher, H. BMJ (1992): 305:1384–1385.
7. Ibid. 5.
8. Fulder, S.J. and Monro, I. 'The Status of Complementary Medicine in the United Kingdom'. London Threshold Foundation (1982).
9. Thomas, K.J. et al BMJ (1991): 302:207–210.
10. Complementary Medicine: New Approaches to Good Practice. BMA: UK, (1993).
11. Meek, C. BMA News Review (April 1993):p 25.
12. Ibid. 6.
13. Soc Sci Med (1990): 31:625–626.
14. Ibid. 10.
15. Kay, A.B. BMJ (1993): 306:122–124 and Crawford, S. BMJ (1993): 306:212

16. Brit J General Practice (June 1992):p 262
17. Ibid.10.
18. Alternative medicine in Britain. Ed Saks, M. Oxford University Press: UK, 1992

Chapter One

1. Atkinson, D. 'Towards A Theology Of Health'. Health: The Strength to be Human. IVP/CMF: UK, 1993.
2. Scott-Peck, M. People of The Lie. Arrow: UK, 1983.
3. Livesey, R. More Understanding Alternative Medicine. New Wine Press: UK, 1988.
4. Gelder, M.G. 'Psychological Treatment in Psychiatry and Medicine'. Oxford Textbook of Medicine. Oxford University Press: UK, 1987.
   and Bowers, T.G. and Clum, G.A. Psychol Bull (1988): 103:315–323.
   and Durham, R.C. and Allan, T. Br J Psychiatry (1993): 163:19–26.
5. Ernst, E. Br J Hosp Med (1993): 50:299–300.
6. John 14:6
7. Deuteronomy 5:6–21
8. Matthew 22:37–40
9. James 1:5

Chapter Two

1. Margotta, R. An Illustrated History of Medicine. Hamlyn: UK, 1968.
2. Lyons, A.S. and Petrucelli, R.J. Medicine An Illustrated History. Abradale Press: USA, 1987.
3. Wiseman, D.J. 'Medicine in the Old Testament World' (see especially select bibliography). Medicine and The Bible. Ed Palmer, B CMF/Paternoster Press: UK, 1986.
4. Coleman, V. The Story of Medicine. Robert Hale: London UK, 1985.
5. Herodotus II.77.
6. Leviticus 19:31; 20:6,27.

7. John 9:1–7.
8. Luke 13:1–5.
9. Larner, C. 'Healing in Pre-Industrial Britain'. Alternative Medicine in Britain. Ed Saks, M. Oxford University Press: UK, 1992.

Chapter Three

1. Office of Health Economics Compendium of Health Statistics. 8th Edition: London UK, 1992.
2. Mann, T. The Magic Mountain. Penguin Books: UK, 1924.
3. Thomas, L. The Youngest Science. Oxford University Press: UK, 1985.
4. Abercrombie, N and Warde, A. 'Health'. Contemporary British Society. Polity Press: UK, 1988.
5. Abercrombie, N and Warde, A. 'Families and Households'. Contemporary British Society. Polity Press: UK, 1988.
6. Abercrombie, N and Warde, A. 'Culture and Media'. Contemporary British Society. Polity Press: UK, 1988.
7. Abercrombie, N and Warde, A. 'Ethnicity and Racism'. Contemporary British Society. Polity Press: UK, 1988.
    Grahame-Smith, D.G. and Aronson, J.K. Oxford Textbook of Clinical Pharmacology and Drug Therapy. Oxford University Press: UK, 1984.
9. Huskisson, E.C. BMJ (1974): iv:196–200.

Chapter Four

1. Harper, J. BMJ (1994): 308:489–490.
2. Allen, B.R. and Parkison, R. Lancet (1990): 336:177 and Graham-Brown, R. Lancet (1992): 340:673–674.
3. Minerva BMJ (1992): 305:1038.
4. Minerva BMJ (1992): 304:928.
5. The Independent Newspaper 5 March 1992, cols 3–4.
6. Minerva BMJ (1992): 304:724.
7. Minerva BMJ (1992): 305:1168.
8. Crawford, S. BMJ (1993): 306:212.
9. Y-T Tai et al Lancet (1993): 341:892.

10. MacGregor, F.B. et al BMJ (1989): 299:1156–1157.
11. Murray, V.S.G. BMJ (1992): 304:11.
12. Morice, A. Lancet (1986): 1:862–863.
13. Gumprecht, J. New Age Health Care. Promise Publishing California: USA, 1988.
14. I Corinthians 6:19–20.
15. Romans 1:25.
16. Genesis 9:3.
17. Nucleus. CMF. (April 1994); pp 17–23.
18. Deuteronomy 5:7; Ephesians 5:11.

Chapter Five

1. Lancet Editorial (1994): 343:553–554.
2. Meade, T.W. et al BMJ (1990); 300: 1431–1437.
3. Kleijnen, J. et al BMJ (1991): 302:316–323.
4. Clement-Jones, V. et al Lancet (1980): 2:946–948.
5. Deluze, C. et al BMJ (1992): 305:1249–1252.
6. Chenoy, R. et al BMJ (1994): 308:501–504.
7. Hall, C. The Independent Newspaper 19 February 1994.
8. Minerva BMJ (1994): 309:350.
9. Murray, J. and Shepherd, S. J Roy Coll Phys (1988): 38:511–514.
10. McBride, G. BMJ (1994): 309:293.
11. 'Summary and Recommendation'. Complementary Medicine: New Approaches to Good Practice. BMA: UK, 1993.

Chapter Six

1. Exodus 1:15–22.
2. Proverbs 17:22.
3. Ecclesiasticus 38:1–15.
4. Colossians 4:14.
5. Luke 8:43–48.
6. Dyer, C. BMJ (1993): 306:1499–1500.
7. Leviticus 20:27.
8. Deuteronomy 18:9–14 and Isaiah 47:13–15.
9. Bury, B. BMJ (1990): 300:617.

10. Kay, A.B. BMJ (1993): 306:122–124.
11. Watson, D. Fear No Evil. Hodder & Stoughton: UK, re-printed 1994.
12. Luke 9:38–40.
13. 2 Timothy 4:20.
14. Philippians 2:25–27.
15. 1 Timothy 5:23.
16. Galatians 4:13–15.
17. 2 Corinthians 12:7–9.
18. Green, M. I Believe in the Holy Spirit. Hodder & Stoughton: UK, 1985.
19. James 5:14.
20. Revelation 5:5.
21. Hebrews 13:5

Chapter Seven

1. 1 Corinthians 10:23–31.
2. Updsall, J. Christian Health Care (1992): 5(1):11–15.
3. Thorax Editorial (1991): 46:787–797.
4. ter Riet, G. et al Brit J Gen Pract (1990): 40:379–382.
5. Reilly, D. et al Lancet (1994): 334:1601–1606.
6. Bopp, H. Homoeopathy. Great Joy: Belfast N Ireland, English translation 1985.

INDEX